The Prostate Sourcebook

Also by Steven Morganstern, M. D., and Allen Abrahams, Ph.D.:

Love Again, Live Again

The Prostate Sourcebook

Everything You Need to Know

THIRD EDITION

Steven Morganstern, M.D.

and

Allen Abrahams, Ph.D.

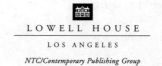

LOWELL HOUSE

LOS ANGELES

NTC/Contemporary Publishing Group

Library of Congress Cataloging-in-Publication Data
Morganstern, Steven.
  The prostate sourcebook : everything you need to know / Steven Morganstern and Allen
Abrahams.
    p. cm.
  Includes bibliographical references and index.
  ISBN 1-56565-871-X
  1. Prostate—Popular works. I. Abrahams, Allen E. II. Title.
RC899.M67 1993
616.6'5—dc20   93-16403
                                                               CIP

Requests for such permissions should be addressed to:
Lowell House
2020 Avenue of the Stars, Suite 300
Los Angeles, CA 90067

Published by Lowell House, a division of NTC/Contemporary Publishing Group, Inc.
4255 West Touhy Avenue, Lincolnwood, Illinois 60646-1975 U.S.A.

Text design: Mary Ballachino/Merrimac Design

Manufactured in the United States of America
10 9 8 7 6 5 4 3 2 1

Contents

To my family and especially my wife,
for we have grown closer in our journey.
— SLM

Why a Book
About the Prostate?

A forty-five-year-old electrician named Jack had been referred to me by his family physician. An enlarged prostate gland had been detected during Jack's routine annual physical examination. When I looked into his face, I could sense Jack's nervousness and fear as we began our first talk. A urologist specializing in "male troubles" soon becomes highly attuned to the emotional state and unique concerns of his patients.

"First, relax," I said. "None of your test results indicate prostate cancer. You do have a treatable condition called BPH, which is quite common, in fact almost normal in men of your age. We will have to keep an eye on it, but you may not need any real treatment for many years . . . and in case you are wondering about your sex life, and I'm sure you are, there is no reason to anticipate a problem."

A look of intense relief, then a wide grin, appeared on Jack's face. "Doctor, I don't know how to thank you. Until my annual examination two weeks ago, I was hardly aware I had a prostate. My regular doctor didn't explain anything to me when he discovered I had a problem. And since then, all I've heard about is men dying from prostate cancer. Someone on the job told me the only way they can save your life is to castrate you. Even when they don't have to do that, your sex life is over for sure."

Five years later, Jack is doing fine and he still has no need for aggressive treatment. Setting his mind at ease with a few facts was as personally rewarding as properly diagnosing his condition. I keep thinking how he could have been spared two weeks of torment if his regular physician had provided just a few minutes of basic prostate education.

Why a Prostate Book?

Jack's case illustrates how poorly informed some men are about their prostates. Worse, many more are *mis*informed. The prostate is not only an important gland all men are born with, it also has a tendency to cause problems. One reason not much is known about the prostate is its connection with sexuality. Although there is more openness on that subject than in previous years, men are still reluctant to talk easily about the components of their sexual apparatus and the prostate is a mysterious one anyway.

That willful ignorance has a steep price. Annually, more than 400,000 American men have surgery to correct prostate enlargement. Each year another 100,000 learn they have prostate cancer. Thousands more suffer from prostate infections and other painful prostate conditions that are noninfectious.

Prostate problems can affect the whole family. Take the case of Bill, 36, who for almost a year tried to avoid sexual intercourse with his wife because of the intense pain he experienced each time he ejaculated. Bill's wife felt increasingly inadequate and in time became resentful and suspicious. When Bill visited our office, he confided that his symptoms had first appeared soon after a brief sexual encounter at an out-of-town convention. That was Bill's only lapse in fifteen years of marriage and he was sure that his pain was caused by feelings of guilt. We were pleased to tell Bill his pain was *not* psychological, but from an easily cured prostate infection.

Rather than finding yourself in Jack's or Bill's position, there is much you can do to promote the health of your prostate. Early detection is a major factor in the successful treatment of prostate problems. Especially as you grow older, you should have frequent examinations of your prostate by a physician specialist. You also need to know the warning signals you can look for yourself.

When medical diagnosis confirms an actual problem, you can do a lot in cooperation with your physician to take personal charge and improve the effectiveness of your treatment. A major reason for our writing this book was to provide the necessary tools to enhance every man's awareness of his prostate.

Another reason was to help dispel the many myths about the prostate: impotence always means there is a prostate problem; impotence, incontinence, and infertility are the inevitable results of prostate surgery; there is nothing conventional medical techniques can do when impotence, incontinence, and infertility unavoidably follow prostate surgery; and, finally, prostate cancer is an automatic death sentence. Belief in these myths has kept otherwise well-informed men from seeking effective early treatment or has caused some to be victimized by quacks.

A final reason for this book is the current worrisome state of American medicine. Consider the pattern of spiraling medical costs, incomprehensible insurance forms, crowded waiting rooms, and physicians who dash from patient to patient. The underlying causes for these problems are complex and their solutions are still controversial. You can be sure of one thing, however—matters will get worse before they improve. Therefore, the more you know about your prostate the likelier it is you'll receive effective treatment. Physicians hate to admit it, but many of them unconsciously spend more time with informed patients who ask intelligent questions, who carefully monitor and record symptoms, and otherwise play a pro-active role throughout treatment.

What You Will Find in This Book

Men like Jack and Bill (and you) will find in this book a systematic and easy-to-understand self-help guide to the prostate. The book should be read by women, too, because they are directly affected by their partners' prostate health. Women can also play an important role during their partners' prostate treatment.

The first chapter contains basic information on the prostate—what it is, where it is, and why you have one. This chapter also describes a healthy prostate, tells how it can malfunction, and explains factors that can cause trouble.

Chapter 2 will acquaint you with your first visit to a urologist. There is a description of the crucial digital rectal examination, the use of ultrasound to diagnose prostate problems, and the promising new PSA test for detecting prostate cancer.

Chapters 3 to 6 explain in some detail the major prostate disorders. Each chapter discusses your likelihood of experiencing a particular condition, what you can do to prevent it, the available treatment options, and things *you* can do to make your treatment more effective and pleasant. Chapter 3 deals with prostate infections, quite common, but fortunately, very treatable. There you may find a clue to the source of that discouraging run-down feeling or that persistent dull pain in your lower back. Chapter 4 describes how your pattern of sexual activity can help or harm your prostate. Benign (noncancerous) enlargement of the prostate and prostate cancer are discussed in Chapters 5 and 6, each describing new treatments that are more effective than was previously available, thus resulting in fewer side effects.

The possible effects of prostate surgery are discussed in Chapters 7 and 8. Chapter 7 will assure you that prostate surgery does not mean automatic loss of manhood because there are effective methods for overcoming impotence if it does occur. Chapter 8 discusses the manageable problems of incontinence and infertility.

Chapter 9 tells you how to spot the early signals of a prostate problem. It describes symptoms you can easily check out at home, ideally in cooperation with your partner, and advises you when and where to seek appropriate professional medical help. Chapter 10 suggests exercises that will help your prostate and your general health. The exercises are easy and fun.

The final chapter provides practical advice on how you and your partner can help your prostate stay healthy. Information is provided on diet, vitamins and minerals, and on avoiding prostate quackery.

About This New Edition

That many men (and their spouses) want more information on their choices for prostate treatment may be seen in the results of a recent Gallup poll done for the American Foundation for Urologic Disease in Baltimore, Maryland. The Gallup organization polled 686 men screened for prostate cancer. These men told surveyors that they were generally satisfied with their treatment and said they would make the same treatment choices again. Effectiveness of the treatment itself was the factor cited as "extremely important" by 86 percent of these men. And 47 percent of respondents said they were "very satisfied" with information they received from their doctor, and many more were somewhat satisfied. However, among men who were not satisfied with their doctor, 42 percent said the reason for their dissatisfaction was that their doctor did not give them enough information. Another 18 percent said they were dissatisfied because they were not advised of all the available alternatives—two important concerns which may be alleviated by reading the newest edition of this book.

Among respondents to the same Gallup survey, about 59 percent of men said they had participated in support groups, indicating that men have a need to discuss their health issues with other men experiencing similar problems. In addition, 75 percent of respondents said their spouse was very involved in the decisions regarding treatment of their prostate condition, which might make this latest edition of interest to both men and their wives or lovers.

This newly-revised edition of *The Prostate Sourcebook* contains information on the latest treatments for prostate problems of all types. Every effort has been made to bring this edition up to date. For instance, the most recent information on the very useful Prostate Specific Antigen or PSA test is included here. A newly-developed medical index for diagnosing BPH is also included, as are new medical developments which include drugs like Proscar, Caverject, and Cosodex, and additional information on new treatment options like watchful waiting, microwave heat treatments, and neoadjuvant hormone blockade. Expanded information on good nutrition and dietary strategies which can help prevent prostate problems and cancer is included in this edition, since nutrition is an area in which new data is constantly being developed.

Also included are updated sources of information which have sprung into being since the second edition. And since the vast majority of computer users are men, Internet and World Wide Web addresses are included in this listing of resources which has been completely revised and updated to be made as complete and as useful as possible to the lay reader.

That Troublesome Gland

The prostate has been called "the gland that always goes wrong." If you live a normal male life span, odds are at some point you will experience a prostate problem. Admittedly, they are not pleasant, but with early treatment most prostate problems—including cancer—are curable or at least manageable, with minimal impact on your quality of life.

As with everything else, knowledge is the key to coping with prostate difficulties. Keep an open mind and I think you'll find the topic fascinating.

CHAPTER 1

The Healthy Prostate—
What Can Go Wrong

Men, try this simple exercise. With your clothes off, stand up straight facing a full-length mirror. Place one finger on your naval, then run it straight down until you reach a slightly depressed area in your groin directly above the point where the visible upper end of your penis disappears into your body. Gently push in—the hard area you feel is your pelvic bone. Now turn sideways and visualize a point inside your body behind your pelvic bone, about a third of the distance between the tip of your finger and your buttocks. Now you know the general location of your prostate gland. If you are a healthy, young adult male, your prostate will be about the size of a golf ball.

What Is the Prostate—
What Does It Do?

The prostate gland or the "prostate" is actually a combination of several small glands encased in an outer shell. The structure of the prostate resembles an orange with a firm outer skin and a soft pulpy center. The individual glands inside that pulpy center do all the work; the hard outer skin provides protection.

All glands are little chemical factories that produce complex substances you need for various purposes thoughout your body. Curiously, medical science has yet to understand fully the prostate's function. It produces some but not all of the cloudy white fluid known as semen or ejaculate, probably its principal activity. Semen is the fluid medium that transports sperm cells, the male contribution to human reproduction.

The prostate may have several other functions. Some researchers speculate that the prostate produces important enzymes or other chemicals. The exit ducts from the prostate lead directly into the urethra, the passage inside the penis through which semen exits the body, so the function of these chemicals should be limited to processes within the prostate or possibly reproduction. In the latter case, substances from the prostate may stimulate activity of sperm, thereby enchancing female impregnation. The prostate undergoes mechanical contractions during ejaculation that may also facilitate sperm movement.

All women have tiny glands that have been called "the female prostate," just as men have vestigial nipples. In their early stages of development, male and female fetuses are essentially the same physically. When the male hormone testosterone appears in the male fetus, the prostate begins to grow. At the same location in the female fetus, however, cells grow more slowly, forming the vestigial female prostate. The female prostate sometimes causes problems, but never as often and rarely as seriously as the male prostate does in men.

The Prostate and the Male Urinary-Genital System

Figure 1.1 (side view) illustrates the male urinary-genital system and locates the prostate. As you can see, the top of the prostate is jammed snugly beneath the bottom outlet from the bladder, directly above the upper edge of the internal portion of the penis. Because space is at a premium in this area of the male body, the prostate tightly surrounds portions of the bladder outlet and a short but critical section of the urethra, the channel through which semen and urine pass into the penis. While efficient, as men age this close proximity contributes to prostate troubles.

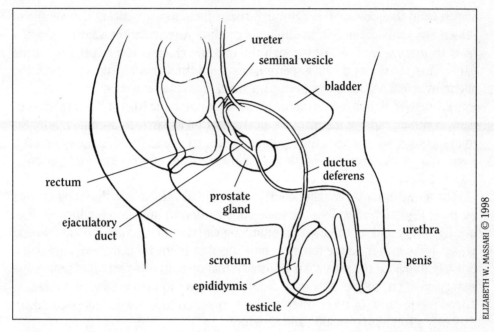

Figure 1.1 *Male Genitourinary System*

To understand what the prostate does, let's trace the path a single sperm takes from its origin in your testicles until it leaves your body. Everything begins with the production of the sperm in one of your testicles. The sperm passes first through a spongy area, called the epididymis. Then, unless you have had a vasectomy, it travels through one of two parallel sets of tubes known as the vas deferens, before emerging into a holding area: the ejaculatory duct.

Up to that point, minor quantities of semen produced within the testicles and epididymis have provided the fluid medium that carries the sperm. But in the ejaculatory duct, the amount of semen increases with the addition of a large volume of spermless fluid produced by nearby organs—the seminal vesicles. Following sexual stimulus and just before the instant of ejaculation, the combined volume of semen in the ejaculatory duct empties into an enlarged section of the urethra: the bulbous urethra.

Not until that instant does the prostate have a role. A separate duct system connects the prostate to the bulbous urethra. As ejaculation approaches, spermless semen from the prostate flows through these ducts supplementing the volume of semen already contained in the bulbous urethra. At ejaculation, semen from the bulbous urethra is propelled through the urethral channel and out the tip of the penis. This journey by a single sperm takes about three months, during which the sperm lives independently, gathering nutrients from the semen.

During ejaculation, powerful muscles surrounding the base of the urethra suddenly contract, causing the main physical sensation a man feels during orgasm. Simultaneous contractions of the prostate also contribute to the ejaculatory process. Even after surgical removal of the prostate, as in cases of prostate cancer, ejaculation and pleasurable orgasm can still occur.

The term "urinary-genital system" implies a body mechanism that serves a dual purpose: urination as well as the male contribution to human reproduction. Figure 1.1 shows that all the internal plumbing carrying urine from the kidneys and semen and sperm from the testicles come together in the immediate vicinity of the prostate. Provided the prostate is healthy, it manufactures its portion of semen, assists ejaculation, and possibly manufactures some yet-to-be-proved vital chemicals. Therefore, because of these interconnections, when prostate disorders do occur, they may affect both urination and sexuality.

How the Prostate Ages

During most of your childhood, your prostate was smaller than a marble and remained that size until puberty. Unless you had some unusual physical problem, your prostate began to grow sometime between ages eleven and thirteen. By your mid-to-late teens, your prostate was approaching its normal adult weight, approximately four-tenths of an ounce. The force stimulating growth of your prostate as a teenager was your body's greatly stepped-up production of testosterone. This male hormone also accounted for other changes, such as a deepening voice and the growth of body hair.

As a young adult and during your early middle years, not much happens with your prostate except possibly a modest increase in size. But during your fifties, your prostate begins a process known medically as "involution." When that occurs, your prostate gradually loses vigor and its physical structure begins to show aging signs much as aging is revealed by sagging facial muscles.

This aging does not mean your prostate cannot grow. In fact, a gradual increase in its size throughout your life is associated with continuing testosterone production—a normal characteristic of the prostate. If all is normal, the size increase will be limited. Unfortunately, in some men, the prostate may grow until it reaches baseball size, or even larger. Then you have a problem.

At this time, there is little you can do or any medications you can take that will reverse or even retard the normal prostate aging process. However, there are some positive things you can do with your diet and lifestyle that may help prevent or relieve prostate problems. These will be discussed later.

What Can Go Wrong with Your Prostate

Too many men become aware that they even have a prostate only after trouble strikes, sometimes dramatically. Unfortunately, the gland is hidden deep in your body, out of sight and normally out of mind. Given its peculiar design and location, the prostate is inherently problem prone. Following are the major prostate problems that affect men at some stage in their lives:

- Acute and chronic prostate infections
- Noninfectious disorders with symptoms mimicking prostate infections
- Prostate congestion—a painful buildup of excess prostate fluid
- Benign prostate enlargement—the presence of a noncancerous tumor
- Prostate cancer—a cancer originating in the prostate that can spread elsewhere in the body

Prostate Infections

Prostate infections occur when a pathogenic microorganism manages to penetrate the outer casing of the gland. The prostate's physical structure and its lack of an adequate drainage system makes it vulnerable to attack. Once invaders are inside, they usually multiply rapidly in the prostate's hospitable environment and make a man's life miserable. These infections can be quite acute, accompanied by fever, chills, penile discharges, and severe pain. Some prostate infections can become chronic, causing borderline feelings of misery and general malaise, similar to a persistent postnasal drip or sinus infection.

A prostate attack can be dramatic and appear to be far more serious than it actually is. Larry and Ann, recently married graduate students, made love almost every day. One evening to their horror, they noticed that some of Larry's semen had dripped onto the white bedsheet and was bright, blood red. Early the next morning, the panicked couple appeared unannounced at my office. In one of my happier moments in medicine, I was able to tell them that Larry's condition was an easily treated prostate infection.

Most prostate infections are caused by common bacteria, especially those inhabiting the colon and other portions of the intestinal tract. Prostate infections usually respond well to antibacterial agents. But it is vital to completely cure all prostate infections, not only to protect the health of the man who harbors the illness, but because some infections *can* be passed on to a female partner. Untreated and uncured prostate infections can also affect male infertility.

No hard statistics are available on prostate infections, but they are common and constitute a significant portion of a urologist's practice. They can occur at any age, even in teenagers or younger boys. In my practice, I have generally encountered these infections among men in their twenties. The numbers increase significantly with patients in their mid-thirties. There is some evidence that men who are sexually active with multiple partners contract prostate infections earlier and more often.

Conditions that Mimic Prostate Infections

Sometimes men complain of stinging or burning urination and lower back pain, symptoms that mimic prostate infections. However, laboratory tests of prostate fluid taken from such patients reveal no evidence of infectious microorganisms. Medically, these effects are known as "prostatosis" and "prostatodynia," depending on the nature of the symptoms. Men suffering from these conditions have told me they've been dismissed as hopeless hypochondriacs by some physicians. Unfortunately, their problems are real and with a little effort effective treatment programs can be started.

Prostate Congestion

Prostate congestion occurs when excess prostate fluid builds up within the gland. One job of the prostate is to constantly produce prostate fluid. Unless its buildup is relieved by sexual intercourse, nocturnal emission, or masturbation, pressure continues to increase within the gland. Prostate irritation, a logical consequence, can be quite painful.

Prostate congestion can occur anytime after puberty and is related to your pattern of sexual activity. Men who experience long periods of sexual abstinence or who indulge in prolonged sexual foreplay without consummation are most likely to have this problem. Paradoxically, occasional bouts of intense sex with repeated ejaculations can also trigger painful prostate irritation.

Prostate congestion can be relieved by appropriate lifestyle changes. Prostate massage by a urologist can also help relieve the condition.

Benign Prostate Enlargement

Benign prostate enlargement is referred to as "BPH"—benign prostate hypertrophy or benign prostatic hyperplasia, another medical name for it. BPH is not cancerous because the tumor that develops within the prostate will not spread to other parts of the body. BPH is however an unpleasant condition. At its worst, it can be life threatening. Fortunately, there are effective treatments with limited or manageable side effects.

Typically, men with BPH experience problems voiding urine because of the pressure the enlarged gland places on the urethra and the neck of the bladder. Men with BPH also feel a frequent need to urinate and the act can be painful and frustratingly incomplete. At night, the need to urinate frequently is very common to BPH patients.

BPH can cause death, although that is inexcusable considering the diagnostic and treatment techniques available today. One case where proper medical treatment could have made all the difference was the death of multimillionaire tycoon Howard Hughes. His extraordinary life earned him major celebrity status, but he became increasingly eccentric and reclusive in his later years. Holed up in a hotel room surrounded by a cadre of bodyguards, he refused all medical attention, despite increasingly agonizing pain from an enlarged prostate. His death was caused when the swelling continued until it created a fatal urinary-tract blockage.

Significant prostate enlargement can occur even in young adults. Men in their late thirties with BPH symptoms are beginning to show up in my office in increasing numbers. By age sixty, about half my patients have significant enlargement, along with associated voiding difficulties. In very elderly patients, it is most unusual *not* to find significant enlargement.

Not all men diagnosed with BPH need immediate, aggressive medical treatment. However, all men with the condition should be examined periodically by a urologist.

Prostate Cancer

If you're an American male, your chance of being diagnosed with prostate cancer is roughly one in eleven. Most men do not die from the disease, though, because cancerous cells often do not appear in the prostate until fairly late in life, at a time when heart disease and other diseases of old age usually take their toll first. In my practice, I have diagnosed prostate cancer in men in their fifties and on rare occasions even earlier. However, the diagnosis is still not at all common until about age sixty-five. Cancer of the prostate becomes increasingly prevalent in men in their seventies, and most men who live into their eighties may show evidence of cancerous cells. Prostate cancer may just be programed into our genes.

If you are diagnosed with prostate cancer, your chances for recovery are good. Early diagnosis and prompt treatment are vital, especially to keep the malignancy from spreading to other parts of the body. Surviving prostate cancer does not mean you will be impotent or have uncontrollable incontinence.

Prostate cancer is almost always a "primary" cancer, which means the condition originated in the prostate, it didn't spread there from a cancerous site elsewhere in the body. Currently, there is no agreed upon medical explanation for prostate cancer. In that respect, it differs from lung cancer, for which there is convincing statistical and experimental evidence of a link with risks such as tobacco smoking and environmental factors.

The popular media sometimes report that an "explosive" increase in prostate cancer and other prostate problems has occurred. And it is true that the number of reported cases of prostate cancer and benign prostate enlargement is increasing. That may be largely due to the fact that more American men are living to an age where there is a stronger likelihood of developing prostate cancer and BPH. Improved diagnostic methods may also be a factor.

Environment and lifestyle may also be involved. As discussed in later chapters, there is some evidence that high-cholesterol diets may be an issue in prostate cancer and BPH. Although that has yet to be confirmed scientifically, minimizing cholesterol intake is a good idea anyway.

Take Charge of Your Prostate Health

Young people are often faulted for thinking they will live forever. By our mid-thirties, however, most of us have begun to become aware of our mortality because some of the more obvious signs of aging have appeared—thinning and graying hair, wrinkles around the eyes, and not quite the same quick recovery after a vigorous set of tennis.

No later than age thirty-five is a good time for you to start thinking seriously about what may be going on in the parts of your body you can't see or usually feel—particularly your prostate. The first thing you can do is to conduct the prostate self-examination described later and to seek prompt professional help, if indicated. Early detection is still the major solution to prostate disorders, so you should also make a point to include a digital rectal examination of the prostate in your annual physical. The next two chapters tell you what you can do and what to expect.

CHAPTER 2

You Will Survive
That Prostate Examination

What can you expect when the time comes for a prostate examination? How can you work with your urologist to make the examination as productive and pleasant as possible? This chapter describes a typical initial visit—you'll fill out a detailed medical history, take routine tests, be interviewed by your urologist, then have a preliminary prostate examination, and, finally, listen to your doctor's evaluation. The chapter concludes by discussing some specialized tests that your urologist may recommend to supplement his preliminary examination.

The Examination Experience

If you're not exactly looking forward to a prostate examination, you're not alone. Most men try to avoid any medical examination because they take valuable time and because nobody likes to sit around a waiting room reading ancient *National Geographic*s. Examinations can also be expensive and they can involve physical or emotional discomfort. And with prostate examinations, fear is a very real factor for many men. Any referral to a medical specialist is often interpreted by the patient as proof of a serious problem. A visit to a urologist for further investigation of a prostate problem compounds these factors because of the highly personal and inherently sexual nature of prostate problems.

Some men's fears may seem humorous, except they are all too real and often of great concern to them. Larry, the man with the prostate infection whom we met in the previous chapter, had an inordinate fear of the digital rectal examination, a vital part of every prostate diagnosis. Larry believed a coworker's lurid tale of the agonizing pain experienced by men who take this test. After he survived the examination in good order, Larry later reported to me that his coworker had confessed he'd never taken the test himself.

Mel, who had an enlarged prostate, semed to be unusually apprehensive before his examination, so I asked him why. He admitted he was afraid he'd develop an embarrassing erection. Although that fear is widespread, the condition rarely occurs. After I reassured Mel, the examination proceeded normally. Later, Mel and I had a good laugh about his anxiety.

In my practice, I make it a special point to anticipate and relieve my patients' fears. A simple explanation of each step in the prostate examination and the reason for conducting it usually allays anxiety about pain or potential psychological traumas. Let's begin with the medical history questionnaire.

Medical History Questionnaire

A medical history questionnaire is required on your first visit to a urologist. Typically, it covers questions similar to those in the prostate symptom check in Chapter 9, but it also asks for details of your past medical history, any current medical symptoms or problems, relevant medical problems of close family members, and for insurance information. This questionnaire gives your urologist information that may be vital as he diagnoses your condition. Never hold back any facts because you're embarrassed or you think a particular factor is unimportant.

If you've been referred to your urologist by another physician, that doctor will no doubt have your medical records. Even so, it's a good idea to assemble your own detailed medical history and bring it with you to your urology appointment. Be sure to bring your written observations from the prostate self-analysis in Chapter 9. You should have this information added to your urology medical history questionnaire as well as to your regular physician's file.

Before your appointment, be sure to find out as much as you can about the medical history of close relatives, especially your father, grandfather, and any brothers or uncles. There could be some evidence in your genetic background that might be a factor in prostate enlargement cases and in prostate cancer.

However, never assume the worst, even when you find a family history of prostate enlargement or prostate cancer. When he turned up in our office, Stan, age twenty-five, was positive he had all the symptoms of prostate cancer. A great-uncle was diagnosed with the disease. I was glad to tell Stan that he was in perfect health. My main advice to him was to "stop worrying," but I also told him to be sure to have periodic prostate examinations as he grew older. This means an annual examination starting at age forty, especially with a history of prostate cancer in the family or if you have had a vasectomy.

Diagnosis of prostate disorders is almost always covered by reputable health insurance carriers. Even so, problems can arise in so-called "routine" prostate examinations. Medicare, for example, has yet to appreciate fully the health factors and long-term savings of preventive medicine and may reject a claim unless there is evidence of symptoms. That should not be a problem if you have been referred to a urologist by another physician. **Note:** If you go directly to a urologist, any symptoms you noted in writing during your prostate self-analysis will help demonstrate to the insurer that your examination was not routine.

Urinalysis and Other Initial Tests

The saying goes that nobody leaves a urologist's office without providing a urine sample. Therefore, after completing your medical questionnaires, you will likely be ushered into a small room, handed a container, and asked to produce a urine sample. Then, someone will record your vital signs and measurements. Very likely, they will draw a blood sample, too.

"Lowly" Urinalysis

The "lowly" urinalysis is one of the most valuable tools of medicine. Besides its role in diagnosing prostate problems, the test is an important means for detecting diabetes and disorders of the bladder, kidneys, and liver, including cancers in those organs.

During prostate disorder treatment, urinalysis helps your doctor obtain evidence of infection, and to identify the microorganisms that have caused it. When a prostate infection is suspected, urine samples are taken before and after the digital rectal examination by the urologist. Your physical examination will likely include taking a sample of your prostatic fluid by prostate massage. The first sample mainly represents the urine present in your bladder. The second post-examination sample contains minute quantities of your prostatic fluid. Comparing the samples helps your doctor locate the primary infection site.

Your urine analysis is usually done in a small laboratory right in the urologist's office. The technician can determine the presence of white blood cells, an indication of infection and the presence of bacteria; and red blood cells, an indication of internal bleeding. If infection is present, material from the sample is cultured so as to identify specific microorganisms in order to assess their sensitivity to antibiotics.

Internal bleeding always means further diagnosis is essential. Red blood cells can indicate cancer of the kidneys, bladder, and urinary tract. However, they might also indicate noncancerous conditions, including cystitis and bladder lesions. Most commonly, blood in the urine is merely the sign of a simple, treatable infection.

Regarding your urine sample, do not make this frequent mistake: Rex was so afraid he would be unable to produce a sample that he often avoided urinating for several hours before his appointments and sometimes he would even drink several quick glasses of water just before entering the doctor's office. When I found out what he was doing, I spared Rex considerable misery. The technician needs only a small sample of urine for an analysis, so you should be able to provide enough, unless you urinated just minutes before you were asked to produce the sample.

Your Vital Signs and Blood

Before your actual physical examination, your vital signs will be taken and recorded. These include your height, weight, temperature, heart rate, and blood pressure. That information helps your urologist evaluate your general health and your ability to undergo treatment.

A word about blood pressure: Some patients who have normal readings when they test themselves at home may have abnormally high readings in a physician's office. Sometimes the discrepency is caused by a faulty home-testing device or by a poor home-testing procedure. Most often, the explanation is the normal tension everyone experiences in a medical setting. Should there be a severe difference, be sure to mention it and have it noted in your urologist's records.

No one ever enjoys providing a blood sample, but it is necessary. Be sure to tell the assistant if being stuck with a needle makes you feel faint. Typically, routine blood tests will provide important background information on your general health. A complete blood count may reveal infection somewhere in your body, including the prostate. Other blood tests can indicate kidney or liver problems or electrolyte imbalances.

The blood sample may also be used for two important tests known as the PSA and the PAP. These tests, discussed later in more detail, may be ordered by your urologist as a follow-up to your initial physical examination.

The Patient Interview

Finally, you will meet with your urologist face to face. If all has gone well, your visit is not quite two-thirds over. We doctors really do try to keep your waiting to a minimum, but sometimes emergencies do intrude.

Information from your medical history questionnaire is usually the point of departure during initial interviews. I prefer to jointly review your medical history and current list of problems, clarifying any vague areas. After that, I probe further by asking many questions, some of them quite personal. I need information on your lifestyle and your pattern of sexual activity. The presence of any sensitive sexual dysfunction such as premature ejaculation provides useful clues for treating prostate infections. What you do for a living may be related to persistent irritation. My many questions about your voiding performance are important to assess possible prostate enlargement.

Of course, it is difficult for any man to discuss such personal matters, especially with someone who was once a stranger. To feel more at ease, ask questions yourself. That puts you in charge and helps you overcome a natural reluctance to discuss these matters. Bringing a written list of questions is useful, because then you will not forget to bring up something that could be important.

Typical First Prostate Examination

On your first visit to a urologist for a prostate problem, your actual physical examination will include these three items: a digital rectal examination of your prostate, a massage of the prostate to obtain a sample of prostatic fluid for laboratory analysis, and an inspection of your penis and scrotum. Depending upon your particular circumstances, the urologist may order more tests, some of which may be conducted on your first visit. Others may require subsequent visits. This section covers the first three items.

Digital Rectal Examination

Despite the advanced technological tools available to the urologist, the old standby digital rectal examination remains a key element when diagnosing prostate problems. Anatomically, the posterior lobe of the prostate is located in the male body very close to the upper end of the rectal passage. When a "digit"—the urologist's probing finger—is extended into the rectum (see Figure 2.1), it is possible in many cases for an experienced urologist, through touch alone, to obtain convincing preliminary evidence of one of the major prostate disorders. If such evidence is found, the urologist is in a position to order appropriate follow-up tests.

For example, in prostate infections, the urologist's clue is a prostate surface that feels noticeably warm. Benign prostate enlargement is indicated by a prostate with a smooth surface that feels larger than one the urologist knows from his training is found in a normal male. A possibly enlarged prostate with an irregular surface covered with ridges, nodules, and hard spots is abnormal and could be cancerous. Fortunately, in some cases, irregularities may merely indicate the presence of prostatic calculi—harmless prostate stones.

Before performing the digital rectal examination, the urologist puts on a rubber glove and then thoroughly lubricates his probing finger and your anal opening. Physicians who are not urologists often perform this examination with the patient standing up and bending over. This method is traditional for men in military service while undergoing the general ordeal of a mass-production physical. A more humane alternative is to be tested lying on your side on an examination table. An excellent position and one I favor is for the patient to assume a "doggy" position with elbows and knees resting on the examination table.

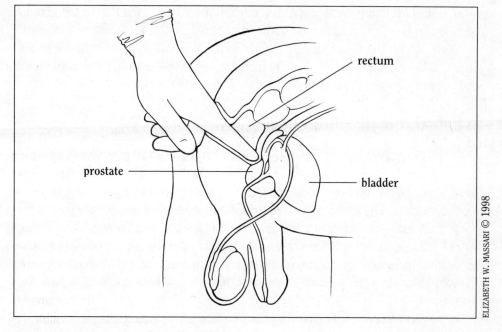

Figure 2.1 *Digital Rectal Exam (DRE)*

Is the Digital Rectal Examination Painful?

Many men, like Larry, are truly afraid of the pain associated with the digital rectal examination. Even more men find the examination at least distasteful. Some physicians who are not urologists do not perform the examination as often as needed, because of this reluctance in their patients. Possibly, they themselves find the examination unpleasant. Urologists, on the other hand, perform the examination routinely.

What is the truth about pain? Authors of popular books and articles on the prostate sometimes dismiss the discomfort of a digital rectal examination as having little consequence. Mary-Ellen Siegel, author of *Dr. Greenberger's What Every Man Should Know About His Prostate* (Walker & Co., New York, 1983), for example, characterizes the examination as "neither painful nor very uncomfortable." To be candid, many men experience only nominal discomfort, but for others, the examination can be painful, especially if a man has an active prostate infection. It can be an ordeal for that patient when, as discussed more fully later, the urologist must bear down upon the gland to obtain a prostatic fluid sample for laboratory analysis.

Fortunately, the digital rectal examination is usually over in a few seconds, considerably briefer than the equally feared proctoscope examination of the anus and rectum. It is much less painful than most dental procedures.

What About Psychological Factors?

Undoubtedly, psychological factors contribute to the level of pain and discomfort during the digital rectal examination and to the feeling of distaste experienced by many men. There has been little research conducted on this topic, but it is possible to speculate. The examination requires the invasion of a very private part of the body. That many gay men practice anal sex suggests a rectal probe is not inherently all that painful. But for some men, the threatening aspect of this invasive procedure may cause an unconscious tensing of the rectal muscles, which impedes the easy passage of the probing finger and markedly adds to the level of pain and discomfort.

It is worth noting that many women dislike pelvic examinations, which are equally invasive. Women, however, have a reputation for being more health conscious and more responsible when it comes to having frequent preventive examinations for female problems. One suggested reason is that women do not avoid medical attention so as to prove they are "macho." It may also suggest that the pelvic examination is less of a threat to a woman's feelings about her sexual orientation.

In men, a condition known as "homosexual panic" may be operating. This term refers to an emotional state sometimes experienced by a heterosexual or "straight" man, who may doubt his sexual orientation, or worse, who may think somebody else doubts it. Homosexual panic is a consequence of a society that continues to stigmatize and even punish homosexual behavior. A man prone to homosexual panic may, during the digital rectal examination, consciously or unconsciously fear that any visible evidence of enjoying the experience will give him away. Under such circumstances, the man resists the probing finger and feels consequent pain.

Homosexual panic may explain Mel's irrational fear of having an erection during his prostate examination, as mentioned earlier. It may also explain why another patient, Lou, was able to report he had experienced absolutely no pain when the digital rectal examination was performed on him by a female nurse as part of a job-connected physical, but he found the examination painful when performed by me in my office. Related psychological dynamics may also be the reason some physicians avoid performing this examination.

As society develops a more mature attitude toward homosexuality, especially as the likely innate biological basis of homosexuality becomes better recognized, homosexual panic will hopefully become less of a problem. A by-product could be lessened fear of the digital rectal examination and better prostate health.

Overcoming Pain and Fear

In my practice, I make a special effort to spot nervous patients before conducting the digital rectal examination so I can help them with sympathetic advice and counseling. One way you can help to avoid pain is to strain downward during the examination as if performing a bowel movement. The result is a much easier passage for the probing finger.

You can also help yourself by discussing your fears with the urologist, which in itself will make the examination go easier. Request a tranquilizer, if you feel that would help. In my practice, however, I have never found tranquilizers to be necessary.

Humor can help, too. Patrick, a highly decorated police officer, whom I have to examine frequently, always insists in advance that he is "a born coward, with an extremely low pain threshold." Aaron, another frequent patient, always asks for a bullet he can bite. On one visit, he even turned up with an empty shotgun shell and made a special point of biting down on it during his examination.

How Effective Is the Digital Rectal Examination?

After all this, the digital rectal examination had better be good. It is, but it is not perfect. A prostate infection still cannot be confirmed without analyzing the prostatic fluid. The urologist's probing finger can only come into contact with the rear lateral lobes of the prostate, so it cannot detect enlargement elsewhere, such as in the middle lobe of the gland, or inward enlargement around the urethra. In these circumstances, the examination may not indicate enlargement, but a patient may still experience problems with urinary flow. When that happens, the urologist may order follow-up tests to be discussed later, including cystoscopy and voiding studies.

Luckily, most cases of cancer occur in areas where enlargement can generally be detected. However, in as many as 30 percent of cases, early cancer will not show up during digital rectal examination in the form of detectable surface irregularities. The good news here is the recent availability of the PSA test, discussed later.

Analysis of Your Prostatic Fluid

Delivering a sample of prostatic fluid during the digital rectal examination takes only a few seconds, although it may feel longer. The urologist bears down with the end of his finger and strokes the gland. This pressure causes a small quantity of fluid to flow out of the gland and into the urethra. From there, fluid emerges at the tip of the penis and is collected on a microscope slide.

In the laboratory, the fluid is examined under the microscope. One sign of infection is the presence of actual bacteria or puslike areas indicating white cells. After that, the prostatic fluid can be cultured in a suitable nutrient medium in order to identify the specific microorganism causing the infection.

The possible presence of blood may also be detected in the prostatic fluid. Remember Larry and Ann, the graduate students horrified when they found blood on their bedsheet after intercourse? That unsettling event, known as a hematospermia, takes place after a prostate infection weakens and ruptures certain blood vessels within the prostate. The sudden onset of a hematospermia is actually not serious and bleeding usually stops on its own as the damaged veins heal, just like a nose bleed does. However, the underlying infection can and should be treated.

Patients sometimes bring up some interesting points about the massage procedure and the nature of prostatic fluid. Mel, who feared having an erection during the digital rectal examination, was amazed to find the sample was obtained without his having an erection. He had always thought that ejaculation, along with orgasm, was impossible without erection. It is worth knowing, especially should you ever have an impotence problem, that this is not true. Greg wanted to know whether he could see sperm when the fluid was examined under the microscope. As noted in Chapter 1, there is no sperm in prostate fluid.

Another patient, Terry, asked before undergoing the procedure whether he would experience the sensation of orgasm during the massage and whether the massage, as a whole, would be pleasurable. The answer to the first is no, the sensation of orgasm takes place when certain muscles involved in the process of ejaculation contract. That, incidentally, does not even require the presence of prostatic fluid, as would be the case in a man whose prostate has been removed because of cancer. Obtaining prostatic fluid by massage is comparable to squeezing toothpaste out of a tube. The process does not result in contraction of the muscles that cause ejaculation, hence there is no orgasm.

Is the prostate massage itself pleasurable? Pleasure is often the last subject on the minds of most men undergoing the procedure as part of the digital rectal examination. Some who adjust well to it do find massage comforting. That may be especially true when it is employed in treating the condition known as prostate congestion, as discussed in Chapter 5.

Genital Inspection

Your initial visit is not over until your urologist carefully looks over your external genitalia, so the urologist can spot clues to your prostate problem. He can also determine if you have any unrelated problems in your penis and scrotal area.

One condition that sometimes turns up is Peyronie's disease, also known as the "bent penis syndrome." The severely bent shape of the penis can make sexual intercourse difficult if not impossible. Peyronie's disease may be caused by physical injury, which was the case with Tony, who fell on a tree stump while deer hunting. It may also occur naturally from the gradual accumulation of plaque deposits in the penis. Peyronie's can be successfully treated, with full restoration of function.

Another condition is warts on the penis. As on other parts of the body, penile warts are caused by a virus. They normally will not cause you any difficulty, but they can be transmitted to a partner. This condition has been linked to increased cervical cancer in women.

By feeling carefully through your scrotum, the urologist can sometimes detect abnormalities in the testicles and nearby ducts. At times, this may result in early detection of testicular cancer. Just as women are advised to inspect their breasts periodically, it would be a good idea for you to make a scrotal inspection on your own from time to time, looking for anything unusual such as a change in testicle size or an unexpected lump.

Menu of Follow-up Tools

Your first visit will normally conclude with a follow-up discussion with your urologist. Depending on your circumstances, the urologist might recommend a suitable treatment program in the instance of a simple prostate infection, for example. When the problem is a benign enlarged prostate or prostate cancer, other follow-up tests will be ordered.

Urologists have a lengthy menu of follow-up tools. Which will be most important to you or even applicable in your case depends on your case. To simplify the following discussion, the tools are presented roughly in ascending order of the burden placed on you for showing up and undergoing the procedures.

Blood Tests

Prostate Specific Antigen (PSA) Test

Since you probably provided a blood sample before your actual physical examination, your urologist may suggest that a prostate specific antigen or PSA test be performed using a portion it. If he doesn't, ask about it on your own. The test is inexpensive, about $50.

The PSA test checks in the blood the level of prostate specific antigen, a protein found only in the prostate. When the level of this protein is above normal, there is a likelihood of prostate cancer. As noted, early prostate cancer is not always detected by the digital rectal examination. The PSA test offers another means of spotting prostate cancer. Early detection of prostate cancer cannot be overemphasized.

The PSA test has been written about widely in the popular press, but it is only one tool in the hands of your urologist. The PSA is useful, but has some limitations. Prostate specific antigen is produced in the prostate gland, and when secreted helps liquefy male semen among its other biological functions. As a point of reference, normal PSA levels are below 4 nanograms per milliliter. A PSA of less than 4 ng/ml suggests a very low risk for prostate cancer, but does not completely rule out the possibility. PSA readings above 10 ng/ml indicate the need for a biopsy, and the possibility of carcinoma. A PSA above 20 ng/ml often indicates to the urologist that he or she should perform a bone scan to see if cancer has spread. However, the intermediate range between 4–10 ng/ml is the subject of some controversy, because readings within this range could suggest a possibility of *either* BPH *or* prostate cancer. In the case of prostate cancer, PSA readings normally rise as the cancer grows, although in about 20 percent of cases PSA readings do not rise even as the cancer grows.

The FDA has approved the PSA test only for monitoring prostate cancer after treatment. A few weeks after a prostatectomy, PSA levels should drop to zero, indicating the operation was successful. After radiation therapy, PSA levels should begin falling within a few months of treatment, but remain at detectable levels since the prostate has not been removed.

In addition to this, many urologists have begun using the PSA as a screening test. The American Cancer Society and the American Urological Association are recommending annual PSA tests for men over fifty, or for men over forty who are in high-risk groups such as Black Americans or men with a family history of prostate cancer.

Despite its promise, the PSA test will not detect early cancer in all cases, including some where the cancer could have been discovered by digital rectal examination. Given the fearful attitudes toward digital rectal examinations, there is some concern among urologists that many nonurological specialists will substitute the PSA test for digital rectal examination in annual physicals and fail to detect some cancers.

The PSA test will sometimes give a false positive—indicating cancer when it is not actually present, which may occur in some benign prostate enlargement patients, because the presence of that condition tends to increase PSA levels. The concern is that a false positive may lead to aggressive treatment for prostate cancer, including surgery, although no cancer is present.

Several modifications of the test have been proposed to make it a more accurate predictor, including age-specific reference ranges. As men age, their production of PSA increases making the upper limits of the normal PSA range 2.5 at ages forty to forty-nine, 3.5 at ages fifty to fifty-nine, 4.5 at ages sixty to sixty-nine, and 6.5 at ages seventy to seventy-nine. PSA results alone are not adequate for a diagnosis, but must be looked at in conjunction with other tests such as DRE and TRUS.

On balance then, the PSA test appears to be a valuable tool, but no panacea. When should you request a PSA test? When you are statistically at increased risk for prostate cancer due to age or family history of the disease (see Table 2.1).

Table 2.1   The Chances of Having Prostate Cancer

Here is a ballpark estimate of the odds of having prostate cancer, using the two most common tests:

| DRE | PSA BLOOD LEVELS | | |
Digital Rectal Exam	0–4 ng/ml	4–10 ng/ml	10–up ng/ml
Normal	Low	Medium	High
Abnormal*	Medium	High	High

A lump or hard area in the prostate.

SOURCE: PROSTATE HEALTH COUNCIL

Prostatic Acid Phosphatase (PAP) Test

The prostatic acid phosphatase or PAP test is an older blood test requested when there is positive evidence of prostate cancer, usually after a tissue biopsy. There is generally little need for it, if that is not the case.

The PAP test determines whether the cancer has spread to other parts of the body. It measures the level of prostatic acid phosphatase, a substance produced only within the prostate. Elevated levels of PAP indicate the spread of cancer.

Voiding Studies

Voiding studies evaluate both the flow rate and the pressure of your urinary stream. Your urologist may order such tests when there is a question of whether a voiding problem is caused by prostate enlargement or by the use of certain drugs, or by a combination of the two. If the problem can be traced to drugs, not prostate enlargement, unnecessary surgery will be avoided.

A more sophisticated test employs a device known as a uroflow meter. Commercial uroflow meters vary, but most measure maximum flow and volume. Some also measure flow time, average flow, and the time it takes to reach maximum flow. The devices are usually connected to a printer that produces a hard copy of the test results.

Some special voiding studies employ catheter devices to measure the flow and pressure of urine from the bladder. These studies are ordered when there is reason to suspect a voiding problem may be caused by disease of the nervous system, not prostate enlargement. Using a catheter places more of a burden on the patient, but can be conducted in the urologist's office with a minimum of discomfort.

Imaging Studies

Given the location of the prostate, conventional X-ray photographs do not yield images of sufficient clarity to permit accurate diagnosis of prostate problems. If you need an imaging test, it will most likely be ultrasound.

Ultrasound

Ultrasound, more properly called transrectal ultrasonography, is an imaging technique that projects sound waves against the prostate and surrounding areas. The sound waves that "echo" from the gland are picked up by a device known as a transducer, converted to electrical energy, and processed into an image. Old navy hands will recognize ultrasound as a modern medical version of sonar, a technique first developed during World War II to detect submarines.

Ultrasound is widely used to diagnose a variety of medical conditions. The images created during an ultrasound scan can be continuously monitored on a television screen or converted to still photographs for detailed study. A typical ultrasound test costs less than $300.

Ultrasound is important to patients with confirmed cases of prostate cancer. As discussed in Chapter 7, prostate cancer develops in stages and treatment varies depending on its progress. Ultrasound determines the specific stage of the disease in individual patients. Ultrasound can also be used to guide a urologist when he takes tissue samples from the prostate for biopsy.

There is some application of ultrasound for initial detection of prostate cancer, although some urologists doubt its reliability because of inadequate sensitivity and specificity. I would never rule out prostate cancer based solely on an ultrasound scan.

When ultrasound is used in prostate studies, the patient must first put up with an enema to clean out the rectum. A small instrument that emits sound waves is then inserted into the rectum. Other than that, there is no discomfort and the procedure can be performed in the office without anesthesia. If you need ultrasound diagnosis for any medical condition, you should find it fascinating to follow the picture as it appears on the television screen. Make the most of the situation by asking the person performing the test to identify your internal organs.

Computerized Tomography (CT)

Computerized tomography (CT) is based on a combination of conventional X-ray technology, computer data processing, and mathematics. To obtain a prostate CT scan, a series of photographs is taken while an X-ray beam rotates around the gland. A computer and appropriate software reconstructs the data with enhanced photographic resolution. The procedure is painless, although the lengthy period during which you must lie perfectly still may be annoying.

CT scanning has been around since the early seventies and has proven useful in diagnosing many problems. In prostate investigations, CT gives a good indication of prostate size and thus is of some value in diagnosing prostate enlargement. It is of limited use in diagnosing prostate cancer because it does not yield accurate images of the gland's interior. At a price tag generally in the $300 to $500 range, CT is not always warranted. Technological improvements could make this technique more valuable in the future.

Magnetic Resonance Imaging (MRI)

Magnetic resonance imaging (MRI) is a space-age technique that only became a medical diagnostic tool in the late eighties. In MRI, the nuclei of atoms generate a magnetic field, just like a small magnet.

When you have an MRI procedure, you will be placed in a small chamber surrounded by a large external magnet. Electricity passing through the magnet creates a strong but completely safe and painless magnetic field that interacts with the millions of small magnetic fields associated with the atoms in your body. The result is an emission of radio waves that can be fed into a computer and processed into a series of photographic images.

MRI is widely used in medicine to diagnose conditions as diverse as strokes and knee injuries. It is being used to a limited extent to determine the stages of prostate cancer. Its cost can be as high as $1,000, and many patients cannot tolerate the claustrophobia they feel when in the test chamber. Interesting research is underway that may make MRI more valuable in prostate diagnosis. At this time, I would hesitate to order the test except in special circumstances.

Other Imaging Studies

Several imaging studies are run routinely once prostate cancer is positively diagnosed. The purpose is to determine if the cancer has spread to other parts of the body.

A conventional chest X-ray indicates whether there has been lung involvement, and an intravenous pyelogram (IVP) checks if cancer has spread to the bladder and kidneys. Because prostate cancer often spreads to the skeleton, a bone scan is usually ordered, too.

Tissue Analysis

Tissue biopsy represents the only way to be absolutely certain prostate cancer is present. You should welcome a biopsy whenever the other test results are at all inconclusive. A procedure known as needle biopsy may be performed when there is a question if an abnormality on the surface of the prostate detected during a digital rectal examination is malignant or benign.

In a biopsy, a thin needle is inserted into the suspected area through the rectum or the skin near the anal opening. A small sample of tissue is withdrawn and sent to a laboratory for examination. Needle biopsy can be performed in the urologist's office and is relatively painless. The patient must be treated with antibiotics both before and after the procedure. Afterward, there may be some rectal bleeding or blood in the urine. Blood poisoning, which is treatable, is a possible complication. Following needle biopsy, you should immediately call your physician or go to a hospital emergency room if your temperature rises to 101°F or higher.

A recently developed tissue test called a laparoscopic lymph node dissection can determine if prostate cancer has spread into the lymphatic system. The test is applied to those specific nodes most vulnerable to prostate cancer. A laparoscopic lymph node dissection requires only an overnight hospital stay and can spare patients the days or sometimes weeks required for earlier procedures.

Cystoscopy

Cystoscopy is an invasive procedure. A rather fearsome-looking device known as a cystoscope is inserted through the opening of the penis. The forward end of the device is pushed forward until it passes through the prostate into the bladder. The bladder is then inflated by a stream of warm water flowing through a tube attached to the cystoscope.

With this procedure, the urologist, looking through a lens at the external end of the instrument, can make a direct visual examination of the prostate, bladder, and urethra. Often, the urologist can determine the specific location of an obstruction caused by benign prostate enlargement, which prevents normal urine flow. The cystoscope also provides valuable data in prostate cancer cases.

Having something shoved into your penis may sound awful, but the prospect of cystoscopy is considerably worse than the procedure. It can be performed at a urologist's office or in a hospital as an outpatient. Cytoscopy can frequently be performed at the same time as a biopsy and TRUS (transrectal ultrasound).

One recent technological advance is the spring-loaded biopsy gun, which is attached to the urologist's fingers and can take small tissue samples without the use of anesthesia during a rectal exam. Also, a fine-needle aspiration (FNA) is a procedure similar to a basic core biopsy. FNA uses a much finer needle and applies suction as the needle moves into the prostate gland. This procedure takes a representative sample of cells, rather than a tiny piece of the organ itself. However, it is rarely used in the United States outside a few major university medical centers because it requires a pathologist trained in examining FNA specimens.

So you will survive your prostate examination. Overall, I hope I have persuaded you that the examination will be a reasonably pleasant and positive experience. This information should relieve your apprehensions so that you can be an active working partner with your urologist during your diagnostic and treatment program.

Rapid advances in prostate diagnosis are taking place. In time, these will lead to new procedures that are more reliable and even less invasive. However, that old standby, the digital rectal examination, should be around for some time.

I also hope your examination results in a clean bill of health. If it doesn't, don't worry—there are many effective cures. Should you discover you have a prostate infection, the next chapter will be of particular interest to you.

CHAPTER 3

Infectious and Noninfectious Prostatitis

If analysis of your prostatic fluid sample obtained during your physical examination discloses that you have a prostate infection, this chapter will provide the basic information you need to deal with that problem. You'll learn about the cause, the symptoms, and how you can assist in treatment. You'll also find information about some other prostate problems similar to those of an infected prostate, but in which the presence of infectious microorganisms cannot be confirmed in the laboratory.

Unfortunately, prostate infections and conditions that mimic them do not receive adequate public attention. While these problems are less serious than advanced benign prostate enlargement or prostate cancer, they are quite common, can cause considerable pain and discomfort, and when neglected can impair your overall health.

Reliable statistics on the frequency of these prostate conditions are unavailable because physicians don't have to report these cases to public health authorities. Typical of most urologists, in my practice prostate infections are detected every day. There is reason to suspect that the number of cases diagnosed by urologists represents only the tip of the iceberg, because many men with low-level symptoms never seek treatment.

Because prostate infections are common and usually respond well to treatment, they are a good place to begin our detailed discussion of prostate problems. Another reason is that prostate infections can occur early in life, even in teenagers, while typically, benign prostate enlargement and prostate cancer occur more commonly later in life.

Some Definitions—
Prostatitis, Prostatosis, and Prostatodynia

The medical name for an infection of the prostate is "prostatitis." Some men refer to the condition as a "cold" in the prostate, and just as with the common cold, a prostate infection is the direct consequence of a successful invasion of that part of the body by some harmful microorganism. Contrary to folklore, exposure to cold temperatures has nothing at all to do with whether you come down with an infection in any part of your body.

Microorganisms cherish the prostate because the gland provides a warm and protected environment, given its snug location and cozy structure. But once an infection erupts in the prostate, that sheltered environment and the gland's inherently poor drainage makes it more difficult for the body's immune system to conquer the invader.

Urologists also use "prostatosis" and "noninfectious prostatitis" interchangeably to describe a condition in which a man shows the symptoms of prostatitis, but where laboratory culture of the prostatic fluid fails to provide positive evidence of an infectious agent. The causes of prostatosis and how it spreads are not as yet fully understood, but treatments are available. There are unproved theories that some prostatosis is caused by viruses that cannot be detected in the laboratory. For that reason, I prefer prostatosis to noninfectious prostatitis, given the possibility that in a significant number of cases this condition may someday be linked positively to an infectious agent.

Prostatodynia is often confused with prostatitis. The term is merely a fancy medical name for a pain that seems to be centered in the general vicinity of the prostate. This condition is sometimes associated with voiding difficulties and lower back pain. As with prostatosis, no evidence of actual prostate infection can be found in laboratory analysis of prostatic fluid. Even so, treatments for it are available.

Acute versus Chronic Prostatitis

If your prostate is infected, your condition can be either acute or chronic. Acute prostate infections typically appear suddenly and their symptoms quickly gain in intensity.

If you have acute prostatitis, you know something is wrong. Gerald, a twenty-one-year-old student, came to our office complaining of very painful urination. He had noticed some mild pain about twenty-four hours earlier, but the condition became progressively worse. In his words, the sensation was ". . . just like pissing with a piece of glass stuck inside my penis." Gerald's other symptoms, all typical, included a continuing throbbing sensation on the underside of his penis and visible evidence of blood and pus in his urine. If Gerald had attempted sexual intercourse during the previous few days, he would probably have noticed something else: painful ejaculation.

Chronic prostatitis falls into the category of medical problems many doctors like to call a "condition." Think of another familiar problem—the nonstop sinus infection. With chronic prostatitis, the infection lingers for a long time, but you may notice only a few reasonably tolerable symptoms. You may not notice anything at all, although something may seem not quite right.

When noticeable symptoms of chronic prostatitis do exist, you may experience occasional mild discomfort when voiding or feel a dull pain in your lower back and groin. There may be some blood in your urine or more often, bloody ejaculate. You may also feel generally rundown, fatigued, and have a general malaise. There may be brief periods when the acute symptoms flare up.

You may even have chronic prostatitis and not know it. Jack, thirty-nine, found out about his chronic prostatitis in a most roundabout manner. His wife had seen her gynecologist, complaining of an unpleasant vaginal infection. As a result of his examination, the gynecologist asked Jack to phone him. When he did, the gynecologist told Jack that it appeared an infection was being passed back and forth between Jack and his wife. He suggested that Jack see a urologist and gave him my name.

Examining Jack, I easily detected chronic prostatitis. He had never noticed any specific symptoms, but after a successful antibiotic treatment, Jack told me he was "amazed just how great" he was feeling. Only then did it occur to him that he had been feeling "puny" for some time, occasionally experiencing a mild pain in his lower back. Jack had passed that off to hard work and the 30,000 miles a year he drove as a sales representative. His prostate infection was probably the underlying cause of those other poorly defined symptoms.

Acute and chronic prostatitis are related. Chronic prostatitis usually follows an untreated attack of acute prostatitis or one whose treatment was incomplete. When that happens, the microorganisms become deeply entrenched in the gland.

Here are some unpleasant prospects: After a single attack of acute prostatitis, you have a 30 percent chance of experiencing a second infection. Those odds go up to 60 percent after a second attack. After a third, your chance of developing a chronic condition is 100 percent.

"Bugs" That Cause Prostatitis

Coliform Bacteria

In well over 90 percent of cases, both acute and chronic prostatitis are caused by common bacterial microorganisms which, unless you have recently been treated with antibiotics, are still present in your intestinal tract. These "bugs," known as coliform bacteria, can easily be seen under a low-power microscope. When urologists use "acute bacterial prostatitis" and "chronic bacterial prostatitis," you can be sure they are generally referring to an infection caused by coliform bacteria.

"Coliform bacteria" are commonly present in especially large numbers in the colon. You may have heard about a nearby lake or a beach being shut down by public health authorities because high levels of coliform bacteria have been detected in the water. Raw sewage contains coliform bacteria and, if improperly treated, can seriously contaminate lakes, streams, and beaches.

There are many types of coliform bacteria. Some types can be deadly as was the case in 1993 when hamburger sold by a fast food chain was contaminated by a virulent strain. The one with the impressive name, "Escherichia coli," often shortened to "e. coli," is particularly prevalent and is the most frequent cause of prostatitis.

There is no reason for you to be alarmed by the presence of e. coli or many of the other coliform types in your intestinal tract. In fact, an optimal balance of these intestinal flora contributes to good digestion. Perhaps you once experienced an intestinal disorder after taking an antibiotic. If so, it was a result of the drastic reduction in the level of your intestinal flora. However, problems can arise if a large number of coliform bacteria manage to migrate to other parts of your body, especially to the prostate, the bladder, and the urethra. Usually, your body can cope with small forces of invading bacteria, but in large numbers, these bacteria can overwhelm your natural immune system and set off a nasty infection.

Other Causes of Prostatitis

Sometimes prostatitis results from an invasion of the prostate by the specific microorganisms that cause the following common and not-so-common diseases:

- Staphylococcus infections
- Chlamydia
- Gonorrhea
- Schistosomiasis
- Tuberculosis
- Trichomonas vaginalis
- Vaginal yeast infections

I listed staphylococcus first, because after prostatitis infections caused by coliform bacteria, infections triggered by the same microorganisms that result in a wide variety of staphylococcus infections are the most serious. About 5 percent of all prostatitis cases are believed to be linked to staphylococcus. Prostatitis cases linked to each of the other types of diseases above are fairly rare, but can have serious implications, too.

The following discussion offers basic information on how you can become infected with each of these microorganisms that can cause prostatitis and describes the treatment indicated for each. Important advice is also provided on how you can minimize your chances of catching one of these infections.

Common Bacterial Prostatitis

This section discusses acute and chronic bacterial prostatitis, whose most common form is caused by coliform bacteria.

How Do You Catch Bacterial Prostatitis?

Essentially, there are only two ways for an infectious microorganism to invade your prostate:

- through the opening of your penis, traveling up the urethra to the vicinity of the gland and entering through the ejaculatory and prostatic ducts, or
- through the bloodstream or lymphatic ducts from an infection site elsewhere in the body.

Coliform bacteria usually reach the prostate through the urethra. Along the way, they establish other infections in the urethra itself. This infection may even spread to the bladder, in which case urine may become a medium for transmitting the disease to the prostate.

Some coliform bacteria can get into the prostate through the lymphatic system, which may occur when a man strains to achieve a bowel movement.

Once coliform bacteria get into the prostate and manage to multiply, the result is an acute infection. Chronic infection can follow after the body's natural defenses manage to contain the invasion, but are not potent enough to eradicate the site once it's established in the gland.

Factors that contribute to the entry of coliform bacteria into the prostate include sloppy hygiene, careless sexual behavior, the use of certain medical devices and procedures, and chronic constipation.

Role of Hygiene

Sloppy hygiene can play an important role in spreading coliform bacteria: failing to wash your hands properly after a bowel movement or after cleaning a toilet or bedpan. Rubin, a young man who was an attendant in a nursing home, was referred to me after experiencing several episodes of acute prostatitis. There was good reason to suspect his problem was caused by the daily requirements of his job—he frequently changed adult diapers.

Carefully washing your hands after any exposure to fecal matter helps you avoid prostatitis. If your job places you at more than normal risk, such as working in a medical laboratory or a hospital, for example, washing with disinfectant soap is a good idea. In Rubin's case, I urged him always to wear rubber gloves, the rule in a hospital, but not always in nursing homes.

Uncircumcised men with very tight foreskins are often prone to prostate infection because an impediment exists to effective cleaning of the penis. Circumcision is sometimes recommended in older men who have experienced repeated infections. Most men in the United States are routinely circumcised shortly after birth, so this problem is not as widespread as it used to be. If you are diabetic, you could have another problem. Male diabetics often suffer from scars on the skin of their penises. These scarred areas are prone to infection and may serve as a source of microorganisms that can enter the urethra.

Role of Sex

Your sexual behavior may be a factor in catching a prostate infection. Urologists report that they tend to find more cases of prostatitis in men with multiple sexual partners. Over a period of time, monogamous sexual partners tend to adapt to each other's "bugs." Men with multiple partners have an increased risk of being exposed to microorganisms against which they have not developed natural immunity.

One surefire way to spread coliform bacteria to the prostate is through unprotected anal intercourse. And it doesn't matter if the penetrated partner is male or female. Anal intercourse, of course, is potentially fatal since the arrival of AIDS, so if you do practice anal intercourse, I urge you to practice safe sex. That means careful selection of your partners, always using a condom, and thoroughly washing your penis and surrounding areas of the body afterward.

One area where hygiene and sex merge is when you have intercourse with a woman who doesn't always wipe herself properly after a bowel movement. Gynecologists advise women always to wipe themselves away from the vagina so as not to cause a vaginal infection. Poor hygiene may also spread coliform bacteria to a male sexual partner.

Intercourse with a woman who uses a diaphragm for birth control can increase the man's risk of urinary tract and prostate infections. Proper use of a diaphragm requires the device to remain in place for a time after intercourse. During that period, any microorganisms present have an opportunity to multiply. This is not a major reason to avoid using diaphragms for birth control, but it is always best to use a medicated vaginal jelly along with it.

It is reasonable to ask if prostatitis should be considered a "sexually transmitted," or to use the dated term, a "venereal" disease. I have encountered patients who are afraid to tell their partners about a diagnosed prostatitis condition because of its possible implications to their relationships. This is a serious mistake because effective treatment of patients with partners ideally involves the partners' cooperation.

To answer the question, urologists tend to avoid applying the sexually transmitted label, given its sensitivity. Their reasoning is that the disease is not only transmitted sexually. Moreover, prostatitis is not classed as a sexually transmitted disease by public health authorities. Whatever you label it, remember that sex can be a factor, so consider that in connection with your personal behavior.

Medical Devices and Procedures

Certain medical devices and some procedures may introduce bacteria into the prostate through the penis. One example is a urinary catheter for voiding urine, inserted into the penis of a postoperative patient. Often, the point where the catheter enters the penis can become irritated and eventually infected. Of course, the catheter itself is sterilized before insertion, but transmission of infection is especially possible in the case of heavily sedated patients with unclean hands, who unconsciously touch themselves in the region of the penis.

Chronic Constipation

Chronic constipation can be a factor in transmitting bacteria to the prostate through the lymphatic system. Straining to defecate can force bacteria into the lymphatic ducts and thus eventually into the prostate. This is one good reason not to neglect chronic constipation. The best treatment for this problem is a sensible diet with plenty of natural bulk and fiber.

How Do You Get Rid of a Bacterial Prostatitis Infection?

How you will be treated for bacterial prostatitis depends on whether your condition is acute or chronic and on the specific microorganism present in your prostate, as well as the presence of any complicating factors. Unless you have an acute life-threatening prostatitis condition (see discussion below) your urologist will not start your treatment until after he completes a full diagnosis, including the results of laboratory analysis of your prostatic fluid.

Acute Bacterial Prostatitis

If your condition is diagnosed as acute prostatitis caused by a common coliform bacteria such as e. coli, your urologist will probably prescribe antibacterial agents of the sulfa type. Sulfa drugs are complex chemicals containing sulfur within their molecular structure. They have been around for a long time and predate other antibiotics like penicillin. Because they have been used for years, their side effects and precautions as to their use are well known to urologists.

Two commonly used sulfa medications for bacterial prostatitis are prescribed under the names Bactrim and Septra. Both are a combination of two generic drugs, trimethoprim and sulfamethoxozole. In standard treatments, either medication is given orally for at least fourteen days.

If you have a history of kidney or liver problems, a severe allergy, bronchial asthma, folic acid deficiency, or are taking the frequently prescribed anticoagulant warfarin (Coumarin) for a cardiovascular condition, don't fail to mention that to your urologist. Either drug should be prescribed only with caution under those circumstances. There is a long list of possible side effects, but most patients are found to tolerate either drug quite well.

Recently, a family of innovative drugs known as fluoroquinolones have been introduced to treat prostatitis. These drugs promise effective cures in some patients in as little as three days. However, longer cures are more common. The fluoroquinolones are remarkable. They cause invading bacteria literally to explode when they attempt to multiply in host tissues.

Regardless of the drug used, you will usually be treated as an outpatient. Generally, hospitalization is needed only when you are experiencing intolerable pain, have a high fever, or demonstrate other complicating medical problems. Other factors that can put you in the hospital include serious urinary retention because of prostate enlargement, and debilitation associated with factors like old age, a serious disorder in some other part of your body, and alcohol and/or drug abuse.

While you are taking medication, you should get plenty of rest and avoid drinking alcohol, which is irritating to the prostate and may interfere with the action of the drugs you are taking. You should also limit your intake of spicy foods and beverages such as coffee, and take a zinc supplement. Foods, beverages, and nutritional supplements will be discussed more thoroughly in Chapter 11. So you'll be more comfortable while acute symptoms are present, an anti-inflammatory drug such as Advil or Ansid will be recommended. When constipation adds to the discomfort of prostatitis, a stool softener may be prescribed.

Your condition may also be helped by hot sitz baths, pelvic relaxation exercises, and moderate sexual activity. There is nothing mysterious about a sitz bath. The word "sitz" in German simply means seat. You sit for fifteen minutes or so in a few inches of comfortably warm water. Your bathtub at home will do. Gerald, the student I treated for an acute prostate infection, told me he put his bath time to good use by catching up on his studies.

Pelvic relaxation exercises are easy and fun. They will be discussed in Chapter 11. As for sex, you probably won't be too interested until your acute symptoms subside. Once they do, my advice would be to ejaculate, either through intercourse or masturbation, because it alleviates prostate congestion, a condition discussed in the next chapter that contributes to prostate problems. Should you choose intercourse, be sure to use a condom so as not to spread the infection to your partner.

Throughout your treatment program, your progress toward recovery will be monitored by your urologist through periodic cultures of your urine and prostatic fluid. The prostatic fluid culture, of course, necessitates digital rectal massage. Fortunately, as your infection subsides, that procedure should become less uncomfortable.

Treatment of acute prostatitis should continue until there is no evidence of infection. This advice, incidentally, applies equally to taking antibiotics for any infection. The acute symptoms of prostatitis often subside quickly after you start taking drugs, so don't do what some men do and neglect to take your prescription drugs regularly, as directed. DO NOT discontinue your medication until you've followed *all* your physician's directions. Unless you take the full course of your medication, you may develop a hard-to-cure chronic infection. If that happens, the unwelcome visitors inside your prostate can develop immunity to the drugs that should be helping you.

Chronic Bacterial Prostatitis

Chronic bacterial prostatitis caused by coliform bacteria is treated most often with the same sulfa drug combinations prescribed for treatment of an acute infection. You must take your medication for at least three months. In persistent cases, it may be necessary to take sulfa-type medications for as long as six months. With the newer fluoroquinolones, cures have been reported in as few as twenty-eight days, although longer periods to achieve total eradication of the disease have been found to be more usual.

The remaining methods for treating chronic prostatitis—anti-inflammatory drugs, sitz baths, patient monitoring—are the same as for an acute condition.

It is inherently difficult to eradicate a chronic infection because it is supported by relatively small populations of hard-to-kill bacteria. Some of these bacteria have developed resistance to antibacterial agents. If that happens, your urologist may try alternative drugs. A second problem is getting antibacterial agents into the portion of the prostate where the infection is lodged. That is a major reason the treatment takes so long. Finally, a condition called "prostate calculi" may be present inside your prostate.

Prostate calculi, or "prostate stones," are hard, calcium-rich deposits that form over time within the prostate. Unlike kidney stones, similar in composition, prostate stones usually cause no serious problems, although they often contain large concentrations of bacteria and serve as warehouses for infection.

In chronic bacterial prostatitis where treatment with antibacterial agents proves ineffective, surgery is sometimes the only alternative. This is especially true when prostate stones are present. One surgical possibility is transurethral prostatectomy (TURP), a technique discussed in Chapter 5 in connection with benign prostate enlargement. Andy, one of my patients, suffered from chronic prostatitis during most of his thirties. Conventional treatment with drugs provided only temporary relief and hospitalization was sometimes necessary during his acute flare-ups. Prostate stones seemed to be the cause. After his surgery, Andy has enjoyed eight prostatitis-free years and there have been no side effects from his operation.

Surgery for prostatitis is not performed on a "routine" basis. As will be discussed more fully in Chapter 5, prostate surgery like Andy's can have undesirable side effects such as retrograde ejaculation. Moveover, unless all infected tissue and prostate stones are removed, surgery does not cure chronic prostatitis.

You may have heard about a recent nonsurgical procedure called "lithotropy" being used with considerable success to eliminate stones in the kidney and urethra. Lithotropy crushes the stones by bombarding them with ultrasound waves. So far, unfortunately, it has not been possible to apply this method to prostate stone removal.

Too many men, out of negligence or misguided feelings of "machismo," choose to tough out the symptoms of chronic prostatitis, especially when their level of discomfort is not too severe. That approach is always a mistake, because chronic prostatitis may develop into painful acute flare-ups. Besides, chronic prostatitis sufferers should realize they are harboring a disease that can adversely affect their quality of life, their productivity, and their general well-being.

Other Types of Prostatitis and Their Treatment

Staphylococcus Infections

As noted, staphylococcus infections cause the second-greatest number of prostatitis cases. "Staph" infections of the prostate can be acute or chronic. "Staphylococcus" is the overall term for a family of bacteria that cause a wide variety of infections, some of them quite serious, including disorders of the heart, the bowels, and bone marrow; bacteremias (blood infections); a type of pneumonia; and skin and surgical wound infections. Staph epidemics are increasingly common in hospitals, nursing homes, and other health institutions. Therefore, you are well advised to elect treatment as an outpatient whenever possible.

Staphylococcus bacteria normally inhabit the mouth, nose, genital, and rectal areas without causing infections. However, they can reach the prostate through the urethra. Poor hygiene and careless sex facilitate their movement comparable to coliform bacteria. Given the serious staphylococcus problem in hospitals, medical devices such as urinary catheters present a special problem in transmitting infection.

Formerly, prostate staph infections were treated about the same as prostate infections caused by coliform bacteria. However, many staphylococcus microorganisms are becoming resistant to conventional antibacterial agents, especially those strains involved in hospital epidemics. Should you harbor a staph strain that is resistant to the usual agents, your urologist should be able to eventually locate an effective medication.

Chlamydia Infections

Chlamydia is a disease caused by a microorganism that can infect both the prostate and urethra. In women, it can attack the vagina and the fallopian tubes. In a man, the first sign may be a painless blister on the penis. In time, a watery white discharge will be noticed from the penis. There may be pain in the groin area. Chlamydia can be spread by sexual contact. At one time, the disease was rare in the United States, but recently, more and more cases have been reported. There have been minor epidemics on college campuses.

Sometimes a chlamydia infection may seem to clear up on its own. If you are diagnosed with chlamydia, however, do not ignore it because it can cause permanent scarring of the urethra, with consequent impaired urine flow. In women, the condition is more serious, because fallopian tube scarring can cause sterility.

Chlamydia is positively diagnosed by a blood test. The same test will indicate the level of specific antibodies available to protect against the disease. Your urologist will then prescribe an appropriate antibiotic, possibly tetracycline or doxycycline. Your partner, if any, should be treated simultaneously and you should always use a condom as long as either of you shows any evidence of the disease.

Gonorrheal Prostatitis

Gonorrhea is a sexually transmitted disease caused by the gonococcus bacteria. The disease, known popularly as "the clap," can cause prostatitis, usually in an acute form, if these microorganisms reach the prostate. Gonorrhea causes a yellow penis discharge and sometimes sensitizes the tip of the penis. Symptoms may appear as soon as two days after exposure, the basis for the legendary "short arm" inspection, in which U.S. Navy sailors were routinely lined up a few days after returning from liberty to be examined by medical personnel.

"Clap" remains fairly common. Physicians are required to report cases to public health authorities. The federal Centers for Disease Control (Atlanta) reports about a million cases a year. Gonorrhea of the prostate, however, is now rare, probably because most cases are treated before the infection spreads to the prostate.

Gonorrheal prostatitis, along with the general gonorrhea infection, is treated with antibiotics such as amoxicillin, ampicillin, and procaine penicillin. Unfortunately, some strains of this disease are becoming penicillin-resistant; in that case, other drugs will be tried by your urologist. NEVER ignore gonorrhea symptoms, even though they sometimes disappear on their own. When neglected, the disease may attack, besides the prostate, other parts of the body, including the epididymis, bones, joints, and skin.

Prostatitis Caused by Schistosomiasis

You needn't worry about this condition unless you are traveling to certain countries in the Middle East, Africa, and Latin America, or have ever lived in a country where the disease exisits. Schistosomiasis, also known as bilharzia, is a very serious disease caused by blood flukes, tiny parasitic worms that invade the bloodstream. A form of prostatitis results when the flukes reach the prostate. That, however, is likely to be the least of your problems, because the disease often results in death from severe kidney damage. You can catch schistosomiasis merely by swimming in fresh water inhabited by the species of snails that harbor the flukes.

Your chances with this disease depend upon the number of parasites that have managed to invade your body. The usual treatment is with the antiparasitic drug niridazole. If you have ever lived in a tropical country, or any country with poor medical standards, it would be a good idea to mention that to your urologist.

Tuberculosis of the Prostate

Early in the twentieth century, tuberculosis (TB) was a major public health problem. The disease, caused by mycobacteria, most often attacks the lungs, but can also invade other parts of the body, including the bones, the brain, and parts of the urinary-genital system, including the prostate. At one time, tuberculosis of the prostate was frequently diagnosed, particulary in men with active TB infections in other parts of their bodies.

Until recently, tuberculosis was essentially conquered in the United States and other industrialized countries with high medical standards. The disease disappeared largely because of advances in public health and preventive medicine, especially the widespread availability of pasteurized milk. Unfortunately, since the mid-eighties, the number of cases has been rising in the United States, reaching 26,000 in 1991.

TB's comeback can be linked both to the AIDS epidemic and to the problem of the homeless. Regarding the former, tuberculosis is a so-called "opportunistic" disease that easily attacks individuals whose immune systems have been devastated by the HIV virus. The large population of street people, as now found in most larger Amercan cities, constitutes a fertile population for the disease; homeless TB cases are seldom treated.

As the volume of tuberculosis cases rises, it is likely that prostate TB will again become more common. WARNING! You don't have to be in a high-risk group for AIDS to contract tuberculosis. You can get this disease by being sneezed or coughed on by an infected person. There is a growing number of strains of TB that are resistant to drugs, and one strain in the New York City area is still untreatable, an excellent reason to find solutions for AIDS and the homeless.

Tuberculosis is treated with a combination of drugs, based typically on medications such as streptomycin, isoniazid, ethambutol, thiacetazone, and aminosalicylic acid. The treatment should be continued for at least one year after the symptoms disappear.

A final point: The mycobacteria causing tuberculosis reach the prostate through the bloodstream and lymphatic ducts. That can occur even during the early phases of the disease, once an initial infection site has been established in the lungs. If your immune system is working properly, the bacteria reaching your prostate are trapped and sealed into fibrous capsules. However, these capsules are potential time bombs, because they may open up later and release live bacteria, especially if your immune system has become impaired. If you have ever been treated for tuberculosis, be sure to tell your urologist, even if you have no current TB symptoms.

Prostatitis and Trichomonas Vaginalis

Trichomonas vaginalis, known commonly as "trick," is usually transmitted sexually and is best known when it shows up as an unpleasant vaginal infection in women. Often, there are no symptoms in men or, if there are, only some mild discomfort is felt when voiding. Men can be considered carriers of the disease.

Trichomonas microorganisms can invade the prostate and cause a form of prostatitis. One reason that it is not common is that elevated concentrations of zinc in the prostate (see Chapter 11) are believed to protect men against the disease.

In both men and women, trick is treated with the drug Flagyl (metronidazole). If you have a partner with trick, or the disease has been diagnosed in you, both of you should be treated simultaneously. Avoid unprotected intercourse until neither of you shows any sign of the infection.

Prostatitis and Vaginal Yeast Infection

Prostatitis caused by the microscopic fungus Candida albicans are relatively common. This fungus causes most vaginal yeast infections in women. These infections can be passed back and forth between sexual partners. In men, symptoms of a fungal infection include an annoying itch on the skin and inside the penis. You might also notice a mild rash in your groin area.

There is evidence that the number of cases of vaginal yeast infection among women is increasing, which raises the probability of men becoming infected, too, possibly with prostate involvement. The widespread use of antibiotics and feminine hygiene sprays by women are believed to affect this upward trend. You probably have noticed the television commercials for over-the-counter medications for vaginal yeast infections. Until recently, these medications were available only by prescription. Some physicians feel inadequate self-treatment by women may contribute to the spreading of this disease.

Prostatitis caused by yeast infections is usually treated by oral dosage of the antifungal drugs Nystatin and Nizoral. These products are also applied in the form of a skin cream when there is evidence of fungal infection on the skin of the penis and nearby areas.

Treating Prostatosis and Prostatodynia

Treating both prostatosis and prostatodynia can present a challenging problem because no disease-causing microorganisms can be detected with either condition. In some 10 to 20 percent of prostatosis cases, the symptoms can be traced to a "plumbing" problem, not to something inside the prostate.

About three times a year, Mike, a patient in his thirties, developed a fever of undetermined origin, and other symptoms of prostatosis. At times, he needed hospitalization. After experiencing this problem for several years, Mike was referred to me by his physician. My examination revealed a scar in Mike's urethral channel, which caused urine to leak periodically from his urethra. When that occurred, the bacteria present in his urine triggered an infection. After I repaired the scar tissue inside Mike's penis with a laser beam, his prostatosis symptoms were over.

When no specific cause can be found, as in Mike's case, the usual treatment for prostatosis involves alleviating symptoms with anti-inflammatory drugs and sitz baths. Various drugs are also prescribed when prostatosis is accompanied by painful voiding. Patients can also be helped by counseling and advice on diet (see Chapter 11).

Prostatodynia patients can also be helped with anti-inflammatory drugs, sitz baths, and counseling. Pelvic relaxation exercises (see Chapter 10) and alpha nerve-blocking agents such as Hytrin and Cardura may help, too. I have found encouraging results by treating both prostatosis and prostatodynia with a combination of the drugs methylprednisolone and bupivacaine. Both drugs have side effects and are therefore prescribed with caution.

Some symptoms of prostatosis and prostatodynia may be linked to prostate congestion, an unrelieved buildup of prostatic fluid inside the prostate. Prostate congestion, which can be closely related to sexual behavior, is discussed in the next chapter.

Helping Yourself—Some Useful Tips

You can do a lot to help yourself if you develop prostatitis or a condition that mimics it:

- If you're being treated with antibacterial drugs, always take the exact prescribed dosage at the proper time. Carefully follow the specific instructions, such as whether to take your medications before or after eating. NOTE: some strong antibiotics, if taken on an empty stomach, can cause nausea.
- Keep all your appointments with your urologist so that your condition can be monitored by examination and laboratory tests. Write down any questions you may have and be sure to get satisfactory and understandable answers.
- Even after all your symptoms have disappeared, DO NOT stop taking your medications until you are told by your urologist that the infection is no longer present.
- Always keep a written log of your condition and report promptly to your doctor any side effects you experience with any of your prescriptions. If side effects are serious and your urologist is unavailable, visit a hospital emergency room. However, that should rarely be necessary.
- Drink plenty of water and be sure to follow all instructions as to alcohol intake, caffeinated beverages, and spicy foods. NOTE: Alcohol can lower the effectiveness of some medications. A combination of alcohol and the drug Flagyl, used to treat trick, can be dangerous.
- Get plenty of rest and follow an appropriate program of physical exercise. Consider seriously trying the pelvic relaxation exercises described in Chapter 11. Sex is recommended provided it does not cause discomfort.
- Treat minor symptoms of discomfort with recommended pain-relieving drugs and sitz baths.
- If you have a partner, involve her fully in your treatment program and carefully follow all instructions regarding mutual sexual activities, such as using a condom to avoid passing an infection back and forth. Be sure your partner is treated if both of you have an infection.

———

Prostatitis should *always* be treated. When you follow all instructions, acute bacterial prostatitis linked to common coliform bacteria can be effectively cured.

Chronic bacterial prostatitis can also be cured, although its treatment takes longer. Some newer drugs offer faster treatment for both conditions. You may be surprised by how good you feel after treatment.

Treatment programs also exist for prostatitis caused by microorganisms other than coliform bacteria. Fully effective treatments for prostatosis and prostatodynia in all patients are still lacking. Better treatments can be expected in the future as the nature of these conditions becomes better understood.

Your sexual behavior can affect the health and well-being of your prostate. That is the subject of the next chapter.

CHAPTER 4

Irritated Prostate—
The Sex Connection

Men occasionally experience hard-to-describe but very real pain and tenderness in the vicinity of their groins and genital organs. Usually these symptoms are relatively mild and disappear in a few hours. At times the pain can be quite intense, lasting for several days, and in some men can become chronic.

These symptoms are frequently caused in whole or in part by an "irritated prostate." This describes a prostate that has been over-stressed by your pattern of sexual activity or, without your being aware, by stimulus of the gland of a non-sexual nature. Generally, prostate irritation is not a very serious medical condition, but it can be emotionally disturbing and can adversely affect your quality of life. This chapter describes how your behavior can cause prostate irritation; and it provides practical advice on how to avoid unpleasant irritation.

There are no statistics on the incidence of irritated prostate. Only the more serious cases ever turn up in a urologist's office. When they do, unless there is a simultaneous case of prostatitis, an examination yields no evidence of prostate infection. Since prostatosis and prostatodynia, covered in the previous chapter, are also conditions where no infection can be detected, it is reasonable to suspect prostate irritation as a factor underlying some cases of prostatosis and prostatodynia.

In my practice, I make a point of bringing up the irritated prostate with patients and discussing the sexual connection. This is a subject patients often hesitate to raise on their own. It is also a subject rarely discussed in sex manuals, magazine articles, or sex education courses. Silence on this subject is unfortunate, given the physical and emotional importance of healthy male sexual behavior.

Your Prostate Semen Factory

To understand how your pattern of sexual activity can result in prostate irritation, let's consider how your prostate normally goes about manufacturing its share of your total semen supply. The process begins inside the thousands of cells that produce glandular activity within the fibrous sheets encasing the prostate. Semen secreted by these cells passes into a large number of tiny tubes and, depending on the individual, flows into twenty to thirty much larger prostatic ducts. These ducts are connected with the urethra.

The prostate in a normal male, if permitted to rest, will leisurely produce about ½ to 2 ml a day of prostatic fluid, about 0.1 to 0.4 teaspoon. Prostatic fluid produced at this rate is known medically as the "resting secretion." This secretion passes without any physical sensation into the urethra and is discharged from the body during urination. If the rate of prostatic fluid production and the rate of its discharge through the penis are in balance, there is no significant backup or "congestion" of it within the prostate.

Ejaculation, by expelling most of the fluid present in the prostate, interrupts that pattern. The amount of ejaculate varies, but a normal man can produce in a single ejaculation up to 5 ml (about a teaspoon) of semen. About 80 to 85 percent of that volume is produced in the prostate, and the rest is supplied by fluid-producing cells in the seminal vesicles, the testicles, and the epididymis.

The prostate is not a super gland. To discharge again the normal amount of ejaculate (5 ml), following an ejaculation, a period of about twenty-four hours of rest is required. Should you succeed in ejaculating a second time within an hour, you will normally produce only about 1 ml of fluid (about 0.2 teaspoon). If you wait two hours after the initial ejaculation, you will produce double that amount. With longer periods of rest, the amount increases until it again reaches the 5-ml level.

When your prostate receives a message telling it an ejaculation is in process, it sharply increases the rate of semen production to a level well above the usual resting secretion rate. This message may travel from the brain in response to erotic mental images or from nerve centers in the spinal cord in response to physical stimulus of the penis and nearby areas. Either way, once the message is received, the prostate produces fluid up to ten times the normal resting secretion rate. This process continues until ejaculation occurs. After ejaculation, if no further attempt is made to ejaculate immediately, the rate of semen production gradually returns to the normal resting secretion rate.

The fluid produced when the prostate is excited has a slightly different chemical composition from the resting secretion fluid. When the prostate is excited, the fluid is believed to have a composition that enhances successful impregnation of a female partner.

Given the way your prostate semen factory normally operates, there are two basic and quite contrasting ways your prostate can be subjected to excessive stress and, as a result, become irritated:

- Your prostate can become congested—that occurs when there is a major build-up of fluid within the gland that is not relieved within a sufficiently brief period by ejaculation.
- Your prostate can suffer physical strain and fatigue—that occurs when your semen-producing mechanism is strained by too-frequent ejaculations.

Prostate congestion is best understood by considering some simple hydraulics. A liquid such as water is very difficult to compress. When more and more liquid is forced into a closed container, the pressure exerted by the liquid on the container walls quickly rises and in an extreme case can even cause the walls to rupture. Should you have any doubt, watch what happens if you try to over-fill a water bed. In the prostate, it doesn't take much of a buildup of prostatic fluid to result in congestion of the gland, with associated irritation.

Of course, ejaculation helps the irritated prostate by relieving the pressure caused by this congestion. It is something of a paradox that too-frequent ejaculation will also cause prostate irritation. When it does, irritation results both from the strain placed upon the gland to manufacture enough prostate fluid and from simple fatigue of the muscles involved in ejaculation.

There is a feedback mechanism operating in the nervous system that ensures a volume of semen adequate for successful reproduction each time you ejaculate. At the same time, it prevents the buildup of fluid that results in painful congestion. An analogy might be made with the inventory practices of any well-run modern manufacturing plant: You always have enough product on hand to meet customer needs, without suffering an inventory glut. Unfortunately, your prostate feedback mechanism was evolved for the relatively simple sexual needs of our primitive ancestors. As you will see, it is not always flexible enough to serve the more sophisticated and complex patterns of modern sexual behavior.

Some Ways Your Sexual Behavior Can Irritate Your Prostate

This discussion will first identify the situations in which your sexual behavior can cause prostate congestion, followed by painful irritation. It then describes situations when irritation can be caused by too-frequent ejaculation. In my practice, the former problem is encountered more often. Specifics are provided later in this chapter that tell you how to avoid or to cope with both problems.

Sexual Behavior That Can Cause Prostate Congestion

Abstinence

Abstinence is refraining from sex permanently or on a long-term basis. Urologists have long observed cases of prostate congestion in certain classes of men who, by choice or necessity, are abstinent. You do not hear the term used much today, but prostate congestion was once often referred to as the "priest's disease." The term was coined owing to the frequent occurrence of prostate irritation among a group of celibate men who, for religious reasons, had taken vows of chastity. These men were also expected to refrain from masturbation, so that method for relieving prostate congestion was largely precluded.

Prostate congestion has also been called the "sailor's disease," reflecting its frequent occurrence in seamen, who, especially in the days of sailing ships, were subjected to extended periods of sexual abstinence on the high seas. Abstinence is also imposed on men in prison. When Mexican authorities decided to permit so-called "conjugal visits" by women at prisons, one justification was the prevalence of prostate irritation problems. By contrast, the approach in the United States has been the tacit acceptance of situational homosexuality among prisoners.

The incidence of prostate congestion linked to abstinence appears to increase with age. Recently, I treated a problem in Willard, a seventy-nine-year-old patient who had been a widower for three years. You may wonder why there isn't a similar problem in teenage boys, where abstinence is still the rule, despite all the talk of teenage sexual precociousness. Young boys frequently experience spontaneous nocturnal emissions (wet dreams), or they masturbate. As you grow older, nocturnal emissions become less common and you may become increasingly reluctant to masturbate. Other factors at work as you age may include putting on excessive weight and infrequent exercise, both of which contribute to increased feelings of irritation in the vicinity of a congested prostate.

Abstinence has become a popular buzzword in recent years. Conservatives strongly advocate abstinence as the best solution for both the AIDS epidemic and for teenage pregnancy problems. In some individuals, abstinence is a moral imperative and those attitudes should be respected. Nevertheless, it is true that the human male body is designed for reproduction, not abstinence. Consequently, abstinence is not natural and can cause definite medical difficulties.

Extended Sexual Stimulus Not Followed by Ejaculation

The easiest way to bring on prostate congestion is to subject the gland to extended physical and emotional sexual stimulus, then fail to relieve the seminal fluid buildup by ejaculating. When that happens, the result can range from relatively mild irritation to something far more dramatic. Relatively mild irritation is probably more common. There is no way to know for sure, because men rarely seek medical attention for it, except in extreme cases.

But an extreme case of prostate irritation brought on by unconsummated erotic stimulation can be frightening. In our initial patient interview, Al, thirty-seven, told me about a painful teenage experience he had twenty years earlier. For several hours, he suffered from very sharp, intense pains in his groin. The episode followed several hours of active sexual foreplay with a young girl he had been seeing. As usual, the foreplay was not consummated by intercourse. After previous encounters with her, Al had usually relieved himself by masturbating soon after he returned home. On this occasion, he did not, having recently read that the practice was strongly condemned on moral grounds.

Tenderness and pain in the scrotum often accompanies prostate congestion. The former is caused by the simultaneous unrelieved buildup of seminal fluid in the testicles and in the epididymis. Scrotal pain resulting from erotic stimulation has been known vulgarly to generations of men as "blue balls," or sometimes "lovers nuts."

Prostate irritation attributable to unconsummated foreplay occurs most often in teenagers and younger men. Older men usually have established sexual relationships or can experience sex without going through an extended courtship.

Contributing to the problem in younger men is the fact that physical sexual capacity and a male's sexual interest peaks in the late teenage years. That is a time when establishing a strong and possibly permanent relationship with a female partner often does not make good sense, given the demands of completing an education and embarking on a career.

Presumably, extended foreplay not followed by sexual intercourse is less common today, if all the surveys of sexual behavior are credible. Prostate congestion from this type of behavior will probably become less rare if appeals for abstinence are heeded.

Ejaculatory Failure

Ejaculatory failure is a special case, when a man is capable of erection and of achieving vaginal penetration for sexual intercourse. Conrad, fifty-eight, often experienced extended periods of ejaculatory failure. During the course of several hours, he would typically achieve an erection four or five times, engaging in vaginal thrusting for periods of up to five minutes. His repeated failure to ejaculate resulted in considerable prostate irritation and caused a serious mental depression.

Ejaculatory failure is not well understood. In some cases, it may be psychological. That can be the case when a man can masturbate to completion, but is incapable of ejaculation with a partner. There may also be a physical reason: some defect that affects the muscles involved in ejaculation.

In some cases, ejaculatory failure can be attributed to a condition known as the "steal syndrome," in which a man is able to obtain repeated erections followed by vaginal penetration. In contrast with Conrad, the erection will not last more than a short time and vaginal thrusting must be discontinued before ejaculation. The steal syndrome is caused by a defect in blood supply to the penis.

Ejaculatory failure is a form of sexual dysfunction not often addressed in sex manuals or in the media. There are no hard statistics on its incidence, but I have encountered the problem in men of all ages. Its rarity is fortunate, because it adversely affects the quality of life and is usually difficult to treat. The condition may come on unexpectedly and go away on its own. Some advice on dealing with ejaculatory failure is provided later in this chapter.

Impotence

An important part of my practice is treating impotence and other forms of male sexual dysfunction. Sometimes, I do encounter prostate congestion in a man with an impotence problem. Prostate congestion itself is *not* a cause of impotence. Instead, the congestion results from sexual stimulus followed by repeated failed attempts at intercourse. Even after prostate surgery, men will sometimes experience a partial erection. These men can attempt intercourse, perhaps with the help of a lubricant such as K-Y jelly, because vaginal stimulation can be an important factor in encouraging them to get more erections. In an impotent man, the prostate usually generates prostatic fluid at normal levels in response to stimulus, but as the man is unable to achieve vaginal penetration, the fluid pressure is not relieved by ejaculation.

I suspect congestion is more common in men who are just beginning to experience impotence. Those who have been impotent for a long time often just give up attempting intercourse at all.

Impotence is discussed at length in Chapter 7. Although the emphasis there is on men who have had prostate surgery, there is useful information on impotence in general. Impotence is treatable and is not an unavoidable consequence of the aging process. Relief from prostate congestion can be a happy by-product of treating impotence.

Interrupted Coitus

Interrupted coitus is a form of birth control often referred to as "pulling out" or some similar term. The medical term for the practice is coitus interruptus. In interrupted coitus, the male attempts to withdraw his penis from his partner's vagina just before the moment of ejaculation.

Although there are no reliable statistics, there is reason to believe that pulling out is the oldest and most widely practiced form of birth control. The Bible mentions how the Lord slew a man named Onan, referring to his ejaculate that "he spilled it on the ground." With the advent of modern birth control methods, pulling out has probably become less common in the United States and other advanced industrial countries. Unfortunately, it is still common in countries where birth control is banned for religious reasons, and among poor people everywhere.

Pulling out is neither an effective form of birth control nor is it healthy for the prostate. As a pregnancy preventive, it obviously fails if you do not withdraw in time. Furthermore, minute amounts of sperm-containing semen normally seep out of your penis even before ejaculation. As to prostate health, the practice can lead to congestion if you withdraw too soon and fail to ejaculate or if your ejaculation is weak and incomplete with a considerable quantity of fluid remaining in the prostate. Both conditions detract from the pleasures of the male orgasm.

Congestion from this form of birth control can occur at any age. I treated Kurt, thirty, for prostate irritation after he had temporarily practiced interrupted coitus for about six weeks. He started doing so when his partner was told to discontinue her birth control pills because of a medical condition. The pressure of a busy professional job kept Kurt's partner from getting a diaphragm fitted. I relieved Kurt's condition with prostate massage. Of course, he could have used condoms during the six-week period. After his partner began using a diaphragm, there was no recurrence of Kurt's congestion problem.

Prolonged Intercourse

Prolonged intercourse is a sexual behavior in which a man attempts to put off having an ejaculation as long as possible, while simultaneously engaging in extended foreplay or even actual vaginal penetration. There are two usual reasons you may wish to prolong intercourse. The first is to fulfill the sexual needs of your partner; the second is to maximize your own sexual pleasure. Both are valid, but they can contribute to prostate congestion. Symptoms of irritation resulting from prolonged intercourse can occur at any age, but are generally more common among men in their middle years.

The extent to which a man is adversely affected by prolonged intercourse varies, but could be caused by differences in the structure of the prostate. In some men, the resulting irritation can be as bad as when extended sexual stimulus is not followed by ejaculation. Normally, isolated episodes of prolonged intercourse will cause at most only minor irritation. The problem tends to get worse when prolonged intercourse becomes your usual sexual practice.

You may be tempted to engage in postponing ejaculation because of misconceptions about what constitutes normal sexual performance. Warren, thirty, was convinced he was suffering from premature ejaculation because he would usually ejaculate within five minutes after initial vaginal penetration. His efforts to repress ejaculation by relaxation and temporary withdrawal eventually resulted in prostate irritation. He seemed relieved when he learned his performance was normal and that the term "premature ejaculation" is correctly applied only to a dysfunction in which ejaculation occurs before vaginal penetration or within a few seconds thereafter.

There is no question that physically fulfilling your female partner is a legitimate concern. Growing awareness of female sexuality and talk show discussions of topics such as multiple orgasms in women have raised expectations of men sexually. It is significant that recent surveys of male sexual attitudes reveal that many active men want their partners to achieve orgasm, despite the popular belief that most men are insensitive to their partner's needs. Unfortunately, sometimes these enlightened attitudes create performance anxiety in men that leads to prostate irritation.

Please don't conclude from the above that I am suggesting that men should not engage in a reasonable period of foreplay and vaginal penetration before ejaculation. But do recognize that extended foreplay, based upon your commendable efforts to fulfill your partner or on your unrealistic expectations of what constitutes personally satisfying sexual performance, could result in a prostate problem.

A word of caution about the suggestions on how to increase your sexual staying power that often appear in the mass media. Dr. Bernie Zilbergeld, in his popular book, *Male Sexuality*, presents a series of masturbation exercises intended to improve ejaculatory control. The exercises mainly consist of suggestions that you masturbate for varying periods of up to fifteen minutes. When ejaculation appears near, you are advised by the author to abruptly cease penile stimulation in the hope that ejaculation can be postponed. While such exercises may be useful when a man has a valid case of psychological premature ejaculation, premature ejaculation is probably caused by untreated prostatitis and will not respond to these exercises. If you try these exercises, keep in mind the possibility of prostate irritation and discontinue them if irritation occurs.

Your Sexual Behavior Can Cause Prostate Stress and Fatigue

Two types of sexual behavior cause stress and fatigue to the prostate. The first occurs when the prostate is stressed by a sudden abnormal increase in sexual activity above your normal pattern. The second is caused by a consistent pattern of hypersexual activity.

Sudden Increase in Sexual Activity

A feedback mechanism in your body adjusts the output of prostatic fluid to the level indicated by your normal pattern of sexual activity. Suppose your pattern calls for sex no more than once or twice a month. In that event, your prostate adjusts its resting secretion rate to a level that provides adequate fluid for the indicated level of activity. Suppose your pattern changes abruptly and over a short period you engage in vigorous sexual activity. When that happens, your prostate attempts to adjust its output to the new circumstances. The strain and fatigue of the adjustment process results in an irritated prostate. A good analogy would be the pain and fatigue you feel all over your body when you take up aerobics after years of little or no exercise.

Two of my patients will illustrate what can happen. Albert, thirty-seven, an engineer, was frequently away from home for months at a time working on important overseas projects. During infrequent visits back home, he tried to make up for that lost time. Each visit was followed by several days of sharp internal pain. The problem disappeared when Albert's long trips stopped.

Ethan, sixty-five, was worried about the pain he experienced in his groin when he again engaged in sex after a two-month hiatus resulting from serious abdominal surgery for cancer. Ethan was used to having intercourse about twice a week. He was afraid that the pains were related somehow to the malignant tumor that had been removed from his upper digestive system. Fortunately, there was no evidence the cancer had spread and in time the pain associated with sexual activity disappeared. Ethan reported very little ejaculate the first few times he had sex, but after about the fourth or fifth sexual encounter, the amount appeared to return to normal.

Such feast and famine sexual activity can cause prostate irritation at any age. Older men are probably more prone to the problem, though, owing to the decreased resiliency of the prostate as it ages.

Heroic Sex

Heroic sex, orgies with multiple partners, and the like, is a popular theme in erotic literature. These performances are indeed possible, but are mainly confined to younger men in their late teens and early twenties. As men reach their mid-twenties, the "refractory period," the interval a man needs between ejaculation and subsequent erection gradually increases. With further aging, the strength of the erection and the volume of ejaculate also decrease. It is significant that the legendary Casanova, who lived to seventy-three, finished his memoirs at forty-nine.

This reality does NOT mean that you cannot have a satisfactory sex life as you mature, but it is more likely to feature quality, not quantity. However, any excessive level of sexual activity, depending on the individual, may lead to prostate irritation as well as other problems. To some extent, the prostate will adjust to a consistently busy level of sexual activity, so the irritation associated with a heroic sexual lifestyle may not be as serious as when the prostate must adjust to a sudden increase in activity.

How Your Job Can Irritate Your Prostate

Prostate irritation may be caused by physical stimulus associated with certain occupations or sports. Men who drive trucks and buses; tractor, bulldozer, and other heavy equipment operators; and operators of vibrating equipment, such as pneumatic drills and floor sanders, often turn up in urologists' offices in disproportionate numbers. Some sports linked to prostate irritation include horseback riding, water skiing, and bicycling.

A highway construction worker, Buck, thirty, is typical. Buck came to me complaining of many of the symptoms of prostate irritation. When my examination failed to disclose any infection, Buck's condition might well have been labeled prostatosis and a possibly frustrating search for an effective treatment might have been initiated, except that something he mentioned in passing provided a clue. Buck casually recalled that his symptoms always seemed to flare up after he operated a pneumatic drill.

To understand his problem, you should be aware that the prostate can be tricked into reacting as if sex is at hand by an entirely non-sexual physical stimulus of the genital area. Because there is usually no erection or pleasurable sensation, you won't generally realize anything is happening. Obviously, there is nothing erotic about a pneumatic drill, but to the prostate, the effect on the gland is the same as when it is stimulated by an erotic movie, sexual foreplay, or some type of vibrating sexual toy—it produces an increased secretion of prostatic fluid. The result: prostate congestion and an irritated prostate.

Not all men develop congestion from unconscious physical stimulus of the prostate by their jobs or from engaging in certain sports. But when the problem shows up, it can affect a man at any age.

How to Avoid or Cope with Prostate Irritation

An effective and rewarding way to avoid or at least cope with prostate irritation is to engage in a healthy pattern of sexual activity. When circumstances make that difficult, you do have alternatives available, including warm baths, masturbation, and prostate massage. Each alternative is discussed below, along with some practical suggestions.

Healthy Sex

Generally, you will promote the well being of your prostate by engaging in a pattern of frequent sex, but avoiding stressful sexual behavior. Fortunately, such a pattern is fully compatible with the sexual desires of most men. Here are some specific points to keep in mind:

- *Frequency*—Studies show a wide variation among men in the frequency of sexual intercourse. For most men, frequency usually declines with age. There are no firm rules, but intercourse once a week is usually adequate to avoid prostate congestion in men at any age.
- *Foreplay*—Avoid prolonged stimulation that does not lead to ejaculation. This applies mainly to physical stimulation of your genital area. With younger men, erotic literature, movies, and so forth sometimes provide sufficient stimulus to cause prostate congestion.
- *Intercourse*—Avoid prolonged intercourse even when followed by ejaculation. Again, there are no firm rules but it is not a good idea to surppress ejaculation much beyond ten to fifteen minutes, even if your partner has not achieved orgasm. Sadly, many men are ignorant of female sexuality. You should be aware that some women are simply incapable of achieving an orgasm from conventional intercourse. If that is true of your partner, consider manual or oral stimulation, which is often very effective.

Men who experience ejaculatory failure despite prolonged intercourse are a special problem. When that happens, you should discontinue intercourse for several days, because the condition may only be temporary. Also, note the advice below as to appropriate use of masturbation in such situations.

- *Birth control*—Avoid pulling out before ejaculation as a means of birth control. There are many alternatives that are far more preferable for you and your partner. If children are no longer a factor in your life, vasectomy can be an attractive option. Vasectomy affects only the movement of semen from the testicles and does not interfere with the normal fluid flow from your prostate.
- *Sudden increase in sexual activity*—Avoid if you can any sudden increase in your level of sexual activity, as well as excessive sexual activity. If you are resuming sex after a period of extended abstinence, do so gradually, waiting at first at least a day between each intercourse attempt.

Warm Baths

Conventional wisdom will tell you that a man should always take an ice-cold shower to cool down after a hot date that ends without sex. Like many supposedly sensible folk theories, that is one of the worst things you can do because cold water can contribute to prostate congestion, possibly triggering a painful episode of prostate irritation.

Instead, a warm shower or bath, including a sitz bath, can help prevent or relieve prostate irritation. A heating pad is an alternative. Some of the exercises in Chapter 10 can be helpful, too.

Masturbation

Attitudes toward masturbation have come a long way since the practice was labeled a "youthful folly" and blamed for almost every human ill including insanity, criminal behavior, cowardliness, impotence, and that old favorite, hairy palms. Even so, this normal and common practice is still a cause of embarrassment and conflict for some men. Despite the reality of sailors' disease, masturbation is still grounds for disciplinary action in the U.S. Navy. And some men, for religious reasons, sincerely feel they must not masturbate.

The consensus of modern medical opinion declares that there is no evidence that masturbation causes any adverse physical problems. Even emotional damage is rare, limited to individuals who, because of their value systems or backgrounds, suffer excessive guilt when they masturbate.

Masturbation has a definite therapeutic role in alleviating prostate irritation. Following are circumstances when masturbation can be a help:

- *During periods of abstinence*—Masturbation is an appropriate choice for men who are sexually abstinent because they have no partner, or travel often. Masturbation about twice a week should be adequate to avoid prostate congestion. If you are temporarily separated from your partner, it is a good idea to masturbate about as often as you would usually have sex.
- *After sexual stimulation*—In situations involving extended sexual stimulus, but not followed by intercourse, masturbation is an effective way to relieve or to avoid prostate congestion. Masturbation is also helpful if coitus interruptus results in incomplete ejaculation.

- *With ejaculatory failure*—At times, failure to ejaculate may be caused by psychological factors or temporary fatigue. Under those circumstances, you may be able to ejaculate successfully and thus relieve prostate congestion by masturbating. When masturbation does not relieve prostate congestion, you should see a urologist.
- *With impotence*—Because of the close association between erection and ejaculation, many men do not realize that some impotent men find it possible to masturbate successfully to ejaculation with a penis too flaccid to manage vaginal penetration. Always investigate and treat impotence. Until your erectile ability is restored by treatment, masturbation is one way to avoid prostate irritation.

Prostate Massage

If you object to masturbating for any reason, having your prostate massaged periodically by your urologist is also an option. However, not all urologists agree with the value of this massage, in which the same procedure is used as when your prostate is stroked during a digital rectal examination to obtain prostatic fluid for the laboratory. In this case, the massage may take somewhat longer because the object is to free the gland of congestion, not merely to obtain a small fluid sample. How often you should have prostate massage depends on your individual condition and whether other symptoms are present.

In traditional Japanese families, wives often perform prostate massage to promote their partner's health. In general, Asian men tend to have lower rates of prostate enlargement and cancer than do Americans. However, there is no scientifically proven connection between prostate massage and a lower incidence of benign and malignant prostate tumors.

When Your Job Is the Problem

If you are prone to prostate congestion because of unavoidable on-the-job stimulus of your genital area, more frequent sexual intercourse may help. Warm baths, masturbation, and prostate massage may help, too. You might try wearing a jock strap or spandex compression shorts at work.

If none of these is effective, you may just be inherently over-sensitive to vibrations. You may have to ask your employer to reassign you, and, failing that, change your job. Perhaps that seems extreme, but the situation is akin to the professional football players whose careers are cut short by chronic knee problems. In the event that your problem is caused by an activity like bicycle riding, fortunately there are many other rewarding exercise alternatives.

———

The sexual lifestyle you follow can be bad for your prostate. Unpleasant prostate irritation can result from too infrequent sex, certain harmful sexual practices, or from too much sex. The practical advice given here will help you avoid or cope better with an irritated prostate.

Prostate irritation symptoms can easily be confused with difficult-to-diagnose conditions such as prostatosis and prostatodynia. In some cases, prostate irritation may actually be a factor that contributes to those conditions. If you are ever treated for prostatosis or prostatodynia, be sure to be completely candid when talking with your urologist about your sexual behavior.

In the next chapter, we'll cover prostate enlargement. No existing scientific evidence proves any link between prostate irritation and enlargement, but prostate irritation may contribute to a combination of symptoms.

CHAPTER 5

Benign Prostate Enlargement

This chapter deals with benign prostate enlargement or "BPH." With any luck, you may never experience prostatitis or an irritated prostate, but it takes exceptional luck for any man to live a full life and not experience at least some of the symptoms of benign prostate enlargement. Fortunately, this condition is very treatable, almost always producing an outcome without lasting or insurmountable side effects.

BPH and When to Begin Treatment

What Is BPH and What Are Its Symptoms?

As discussed in Chapter 1, two medical terms refer to benign enlargement of the prostate: "benign prostatic hypertrophy" and "benign prostate hyperplasia." The second is more recent and is increasingly preferred by urologists. It is too bad "BPH" stands for both, because that causes needless confusion.

"Hypertrophy" is a fancy word that means the excessive and undesirable development of any body organ or part. "Hyperplasia" means an abnormal increase in the number of cells that causes enlargment in the affected body organ or part.

When used in medicine, "benign" means not malignant—not cancerous. A malignant or cancerous tumor is an abnormal growth that can spread from its site of origin inside the body to other, often distant, parts of the body. A benign tumor, on the other hand, will not spread and will usually not recur once it is completely removed surgically. You should be aware, however, that a benign prostate tumor is anything but benign in the sense that the word is used in everyday speech as something kindly, gentle, or mild. In 1990, approximately four hundred American men died from complications of BPH. Most deaths were brought on by acute urinary retention followed by kidney failure. Fortunately, there is good news—in 1970, with a significantly smaller national population, there were about 2,200 deaths, almost six times more than twenty years later. Obviously, encouraging progress is being made in detection and timely treatment of severe cases of BPH.

BPH first appears when a mass of glandular tissue, known medically as an adenoma, begins to form on a base of normal prostatic tissue. Usually, this tissue growth begins initially in the two lateral and median lobes of the prostate (see Figure 5.1). Growth is usually inward toward the urethral channel, which commonly creates pressure on the urethra causing reduced urine flow. When that happens, the symptoms include a frequent need to urinate (especially at night), extended hesitation before the appearance of your urinary stream, a weak or intermittent urinary stream, and a feeling after you finish that your bladder has not emptied completely. The checklist in Chapter 9 will help you recognize and evaluate voiding symptoms.

There is some evidence that the enlarged prostate pressing on the urethra is not the only factor affecting voiding. Some men with considerably enlarged prostates experience only minimal voiding difficulties, while others with only minor enlargement experience severe symptoms. In any event, symptoms may wax or wane in intensity, often getting worse after exposure to cold, to alcohol, or to some drugs. Medical research suggests damage to the smooth muscles of the bladder may occur as the prostate tumor increases the obstruction and irritation in the vicinity of the bladder neck. As tissues deteriorate, the smooth bladder muscles are subjected to cycles of uncontrolled expansion and contraction, resulting in episodes of voiding urgency and even urinary incontinence.

While benign prostate growth can begin in some men as early as age thirty, in most cases significant growth, along with noticeable voiding symptoms, do not take place until the middle years. After symptoms are first noticed, they tend to increase gradually in frequency and intensity, although there is no set pattern. The disease is at an advanced stage and becomes increasingly life threatening when painful retention of urine in the bladder becomes frequent. This stage coincides with potentially serious damage to the smooth bladder muscles.

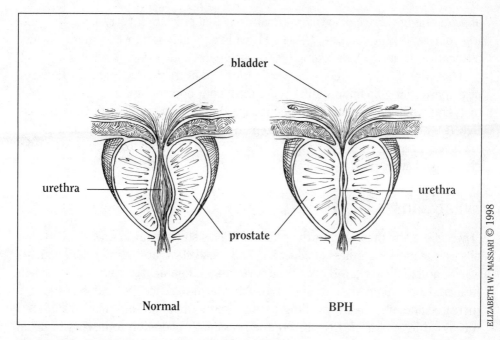

Figure 5.1 *Benign Prostatic Hyperplasia (BPH)*

BPH and other prostate conditions can be diagnosed by closely examining a patient's urinary habits. Therefore, patients are often asked to keep a record or log of their urinary habits, writing down any symptoms or problems and when they occur. This log provides more detailed information, and it can help a urologist assess a patient's symptoms. Because not every urologist asks the same questions, or receives identical answers, the American Urological Association has standardized this process by devising a short checklist of symptoms to determine the likelihood of BPH, (see Apppendix E).

Your BPH Odds

Unless you had the obvious misfortune of being castrated as a child, your odds are not very good for avoiding BPH, even in a mild form, as you age. About half of all men by age sixty, and 90 percent by age eighty experience some degree of BPH. In most instances, the condition is fairly mild. Nevertheless, by age fifty, you have about a one-in-three chance of eventually needing prostate surgery sometime during your remaining lifetime. These odds will very likely improve as more effective alternatives to surgery, including new drugs, become increasingly available.

Over 400,000 BPH operations were performed in the United States in 1990 at a cost approaching $5 billion. BPH is the most common condition treated by urologists and reportedly accounts for about a third of a typical urologist's clinical practice. It is also one of the most common men's diseases paid for by Medicare.

It has never been proven that having BPH either increases or decreases your chances of having prostate cancer.

What Causes BPH?

There are many theories, but the cause of BPH is still a medical mystery. It strikes all types of men, regardless of education and social class: one of my recent patients was a sanitation worker. By contrast, a recent well-publicized case was President Reagan, who had prostate surgery during his term in office. Indicative of society's increased and more healthy willingness to discuss what had been a taboo subject, I was asked to appear on CNN before the president's operation to discuss in detail the surgical procedure.

No convincing evidence links a history of prostatitis or any particular pattern of sexual behavior to the disease. There is also no confirmed evidence of a link to environmental factors or to racial or ethnic heritage, except for the single exception of Asian men, discussed below. According to a recent study conducted at Johns Hopkins University, a small percentage of men—perhaps 7 percent—have a gene which makes them more inclined to BPH. Men who get BPH at a younger age seem more likely to carry this gene.

BPH is somehow related both to age and to the level of testosterone in the bloodstream. An early clue for medical researchers was their observation that BPH was virtually unknown among the palace eunuchs of vanished Chinese and Ottoman Empires, regardless of age. These men, of course, had minimal testosterone levels.

Testosterone is a steroid-type hormone produced mainly in the testicles and to a lesser extent in the adrenal glands, so some will still be present even after castration. Testosterone is essential to the normal development of a male fetus, because it is the substance that triggers and drives the biological processes that cause development of male sexual organs. Later, testosterone is the male sex hormone essential to the changes that occur in boys during puberty, including enlargement of the prostate gland to the size characteristic of a young adult. Still later, a certain amount of testosterone is needed to sustain adequate sexual performance and physical vigor in the male body.

Testosterone output in most men begins to increase at puberty and continues to rise until it peaks in the mid to late thirties. At that point, it slowly declines. In some men, insufficient testosterone causes declining sexual performance and flagging sexual interest (libido). These men may benefit from carefully monitored testosterone supplements. Unfortunately, in some men, even a declining rate of production still provides too much testosterone, resulting in the growth of a benign prostate tumor.

It may be that the evolutionary process in early man programmed into their DNA an effective mechanism by which testosterone "turns on" the desired growth of the prostate at puberty, but has no consequent mechanism to "turn off" growth after the gland reaches its adult size. If that theory is correct, there will be continued growth of the prostate, regardless of undesirable consequences and despite diminishing testosterone. It may be that reproduction is more essential to the survival of the species than the comfort or even the lifespan of older males, and we simply suffer from a built-in problem.

There is some reason to believe that the old menace cholesterol may play a role in BPH. Cholesterol is also a steroid substance with a chemical structure bearing certain similarities to testosterone. It is well established that Asian men tend to have a lower incidence of BPH than Americans. Asians traditionally eat food lower in cholesterol—rice and noodles, lots of vegetables, and smaller amounts of meat and fish, added to their diets mainly for seasoning. There is also minimal fat in an Asian diet and even then, fat is often in the form of fish oils. Men of Asian extraction living in the United States who eat a typical American artery-plugging fast-food diet suffer from BPH at levels comparable to other Americans, suggesting that there is no genetic factor based solely upon racial characteristics.

Both the prostate tissues and prostatic fluid are high in naturally-occurring cholesterol. Various theories have suggested a mechanism by which bad diet may promote benign tumor growth by loading the prostate with excess cholesterol. The jury is still out on that idea. In one recent study, a high-cholesterol diet failed to cause BPH in rats. Other recent studies have shown some possible beneficial impact on BPH from cholesterol-lowering drugs. I am inclined to think excess cholesterol *is* a factor in BPH, but regardless of the ultimate findings, you are well advised to minimize cholesterol intake for other good reasons, most importantly, your cardiovascular health.

It is interesting that man and his best friend, the dog, are the only mammalian species that suffer from BPH. Many animals, including rats and various species of monkeys, have prostates but never experience BPH. The availability of dogs for BPH research by urologists and veterinarians has helped develop improved surgical and nonsurgical treatment to the mutual benefit of both species.

When Should BPH Be Treated?

The consensus among urologists is that aggressive treatment of BPH can be postponed until just before the point when there is a real possibility of bladder and kidney damage, or when the condition has progressed to an unacceptable level of inconvenience and discomfort to the patient. This approach emphasizes careful monitoring of the condition by periodic examination. Despite a tendency to "push" prostate surgery, especially among Medicare and other insured patients, there is no evidence that the vast majority of urologists needlessly encourage premature or unnecessary treatment. Should you have any doubts in your own case, don't hesitate to get a second opinion. In fact, second opinions are mandatory under some insurance programs.

Putting off aggressive treatment, especially surgery, is sensible. Nobody ever wants to have surgery and it is possible, given the accelerating pace of development in alternative BPH treatments, that putting it off for just the next few years may result in the appearance of a new treatment that may make surgery unnecessary for you.

However, there are two basic problems in putting off treatment: You must be absolutely certain the disease does not progress to the point where it causes bladder and kidney damage. The second is deciding what level of inconvenience and discomfort is unacceptable for you.

Kidney and Bladder Damage

Bad news: There is no way to predict how long it takes from the onset of symptoms until they reach the point where there is a possibility of kidney or bladder damage. While BPH symptoms tend to worsen over time, the progress of the disease is often characterized by static periods when there is little change in symptoms and others when symptoms are noticeably worse. Each patient is unique.

Sometimes the course of BPH is characterized by a condition known as "silent BPH," which occurs when gland growth takes place that does not result in direct pressure on the urethra. In that event, the usual voiding symptoms of BPH may not be obvious and may be absent altogether. However, bladder and kidney damage may still be possible.

Silent BPH may cause hemorrhoids when the gland expands toward the rectum. However, hemorrhoids are fairly common, so an examining physician may overlook the possibility that their presence signals a deteriorating BPH condition. All too often, the first awareness of a serious problem with silent BPH may not occur until the sufferer ends up in a hospital emergency room with a painful episode of urine retention. These emergencies often occur after significant alcohol consumption or exposure to severe cold temperatures. These factors can themselves create urinary retention by triggering involuntary smooth muscle contractions at the bladder neck.

Conditions such as recurring and often serious urinary tract infections, stones, diverticula (pouches in the bladder wall), and sometimes high blood pressure, frequently accompany and can be possible symptoms of damage to the smooth muscles of the bladder. When these conditions occur, your urologist should consider silent BPH, even in the absence of serious voiding symptoms, or any evidence of enlargement during a digital rectal examination.

Blood in the urine and painful ejaculation are two powerful signals that you need aggressive treatment, even if you feel that you can live with voiding problems. You may find blood in your urine if you're suffering from BPH, because the blood vessels supplying your prostate are forced to deliver additional blood to supply the increased volume the enlarged gland needs to maintain its cellular activity. When the vessels become overloaded well beyond their capacity, they can rupture and leak. While this bleeding is not especially serious, it does indicate the disease has advanced significantly. NEVER IGNORE blood in your urine, because its presence could signal a far more serious condition than mere BPH.

When an enlarged prostate gland impinges on the urethra, a man may feel considerable pain when he ejaculates. However, the most common reason for painful ejaculation is a prostate infection. If there's no evidence of infection or if appropriate treatment brings no relief for voiding symptoms, then benign prostate enlargement is probably the cause and is approaching the stage at which aggressive treatment may be needed.

Today, there is no excuse for any man to let BPH remain untreated until it becomes fatal due to bladder rupture or urine backup into the kidney with deadly kidney malfunction. There was certainly no excuse in Howard Hughes's case. He could obviously afford the best medical care, as we mentioned in Chapter 1. Most of the roughly four hundred or so annual deaths from BPH that occur in the United States are probably poor men, who have no access to adequate medical treatment, or other men who decline medical treatment on religious grounds.

When Do BPH Symptoms Become Unacceptable?

An "acceptable" level of inconvenience and discomfort is a highly subjective one that varies with each patient. Frequent urination is more of a problem for university professors giving two-hour lectures than for office workers whose work stations are close to the men's room. Men who travel often, trapped for lengthy periods on airplanes with the seat belt sign lit, have special problems, too. Furthermore, some men are more tolerant of the discomfort. Age is also a factor, particularly in older men in poor health who may be poor risks for surgery, but who are not immediate prospects for severe bladder or kidney damage.

One of my more interesting cases was Jason, fifty-four, a university basketball coach. He tolerated his voiding symptoms reasonably well for about five years. But toward the end of that period it became more difficult to get through an evening's coaching. As any basketball fan is aware, the coach is highly visible on the floor during the entire game, usually agonizing over his team's progress. There are few opportunities for frequent quick trips to the men's room. Jason decided his treatment could not wait. He opted for a successful balloon dilatation, which is discussed below. If Jason had been the manager of a baseball team, less visible in the dugout and more convenient to the locker room, he might have held out a little longer before opting for treatment.

It is always better, I feel, to start aggressive treatment sooner rather than later, not only to avoid bladder or kidney damage, but to improve the patient's quality of life. I have had many patients, such as Dale, a forty-eight-year-old journalist, who put off treatment too long and later, after enjoying the relief, regretted not doing something sooner. There is some analogy to putting off treatment of BPH to wearing a truss for a hernia instead of having that condition repaired properly in order to return to a more active life.

Treating BPH with Surgery

Traditional Surgical Treatments

The earliest surgical treatment for BPH was drastic and not always effective—castration. However, this operation became fairly common over a hundred years ago when the link between testosterone and prostate enlargement first became generally understood. Orchiectomy, the medical term for surgical removal of the testicles, gradually fell out of favor when surgical procedures began for removing excess prostate tissue. Today, castration as a treatment for BPH is very rare, but is still practiced to some extent in some cases of prostate cancer, as we will see in the next chapter.

During the late nineteenth century, two "open" surgical procedures were developed for removing both benign and malignant prostate tissue: perineal and suprapubic prostatectomy. Perineal prostatectomies, involving an incision through the crotch about halfway between the scrotum and anus are rarely used today to treat BPH. The awkward position the procedure requires is a burden on older patients. There is also an increased possibility of rectal injury. Perineal prostatectomies are performed in certain cases of prostate cancer by veteran urologists who are more familiar with the procedure.

Suprapubic prostatectomy, described below, is principally performed nowadays in special situations and in relatively few institutions. The main reasons it is performed at all is because it is quick and does not require the skill level of other procedures.

A more common open procedure known as retropubic prostatectomy appeared in the mid-forties. Transurethral prostatectomy (TURP), a "closed" procedure, came into practice about the same time. If you need BPH surgery, a TURP will likely be your choice.

Suprapubic Prostatectomy

Suprapubic prostatectomy is called an "open" operation because a surgical incision is made into the body. In any open operation, it is implicit that an exposed wound is created that may cause pain and possibly complicate recovery. However, an open prostatectomy may be the best choice when the gland is greatly enlarged so that a "closed" procedure, discussed below, is precluded.

In suprapubic prostatectomies, an incision is made in the pubic area of the lower abdomen a few inches above the point where the penis enters the body.

Continuing this opening into the bladder, the urologist can reach the top of the prostate by extending his instruments through the bladder. The surgeon can then cut out and remove excess prostate tissue. This operation usually requires two drainage catheters, which typically remain in place for about a week while the patient recovers.

The main advantage of a suprapubic prostatectomy is that the urologist has direct access to the interior of the bladder. He can examine it, easily remove any stones, and repair any pouches he finds in the bladder wall. There is less chance of impotence than with perineal prostatectomy, although not all researchers agree with that judgment. The disadvantages include considerable bleeding, the damage to the bladder, and that the operation is relatively tough on the patient, requiring a lengthy hospital stay. These patients are usually hospitalized from ten days to two weeks and are unable to return to work for about a month.

Retropubic Prostatectomy

In a retropubic prostatectomy, the urologist makes an incision through the abdomen in the same location as in a suprapubic prostatectomy, but he carefully extends the incision along the front of the bladder to completely bypass it. He extends the incision further and enters the prostate from the front, from which point he can remove all the excess prostate tissue.

One important advantage: The retropubic prostatectomy lets the urologist take a good look at the prostate by direct visual inspection of the gland's condition, which facilitates surgical removal of excess tissue. There is less blood loss than with a suprapubic prostatectomy and only a single drainage catheter is needed and that for a shorter period of time. Patients go home and back to work after much briefer periods. Consequently, retropubic prostatectomies have largely supplanted suprapubic prostatectomies. One exception is when patients need simultaneous treatment for known bladder problems.

Transurethral Resection (TURP)

Urologists sometimes refer to transurethral resection as the "roto-rooter" method, because of its similarity to the pipe cleaning system used by plumbers. TURP is a closed procedure that does not involve a surgical incision and was the procedure employed to treat President Reagan's prostate problem. Given its advantages, TURPs account for about 90 percent of all prostatectomies for benign prostate enlargement.

In a TURP, the urologist uses an operating instrument known as a resectoscope, similar to the cystoscope used to inspect the urethra and bladder. The tip of the resectoscope is inserted into the opening of the penis and passed through the previously well-lubricated urethral channel and stopped when the tip of the instrument enters the bladder. With proper medication, the procedure is easily tolerated by the patient.

Once the instrument is in place, the urologist looks through the resectoscope and studies the obstruction caused by the enlarged prostate to determine if there are other complications, such as a bladder tumor. If all is well, the urologist leaves the resectoscope in place and uses surgical intruments incorporated in the device to remove excess tissue obstructing urine flow through the urethra. Should there be any complications, the urologist may remove the instrument and perform an open prostatectomy.

An electrically charged fine circular wire known as a "hot loop" is used most often to cut away excess prostate tissue. During the procedure, the area being cut away is lubricated by a flow of distilled water or a dilute solution of glycine. This irrigating stream is warmed to normal body temperature. The cutting produces small bits of tissue that initially accumulate inside the bladder. As the procedure progresses, these bits are washed out of the body from time to time by an irrigating stream of water.

Today, two other removal techniques are available. The "cold punch" method uses a hollow circular knife instead of a hot loop. There is little difference and no really strong advantages between these techniques. Urologists use one or the other depending on their training.

The second is cryogenic cutting in which a stream of liquid nitrogen, cooled to minus 180° C (minus 356° F), is passed through the resectoscope. The liquid nitrogen freezes and so kills excess prostate tissue. The resectoscope is removed after the tissue is frozen and a catheter is inserted through the urethra. In a few days, dead tissue begins to slough off, passing out through the catheter.

Cryogenic cutting is quick and causes less blood loss. Its principal disadvantage is that current technology does not permit adequate control of the frozen tissue area, so that removal of excess tissue may be insufficient. There may also be damage to the rectum and nearby tissue. A lengthy period of catheter drainage is also required and problems can arise during removal of large bits of dead tissue. Thus, despite its promise, cryogenic cutting is an experimental procedure, and limited to a few patient volunteers.

Transurethral resection has important advantages; it can almost always be performed in less than an hour and typically requires only a three- to five-day hospital stay. No abdominal incision is needed, so it is less painful than open prostatectomy and there are fewer surgical complications. TURP undergoes constant improvements. Some urologists already use television cameras to monitor the course of the operation, providing an enlarged and clearer view of the prostate region and eliminating the need for the urologist to squint with one eye through the resectoscope during surgery.

Nevertheless, TURP has its downside, too. As indicated previously, a suprapubic prostatectomy may be preferable when a patient has problems with bladder stones or pouches. There can also be problems when treating patients with greatly enlarged prostates. The time and the strain of the surgical procedure increases proportionally with the gland's size. Most urologists prefer not to perform a TURP that will take longer than an hour and, as an alternative, will suggest an open prostatectomy. However, many TURPs are performed in healthy patients for periods up to two hours.

Urologists also disagree about the long-term effects of transurethral resection, compared with open prostatectomy. Some evidence suggests open prostatectomies do a more thorough job of removing urinary obstructions and thus need follow-up surgery less often. Your chances of needing a second operation after having a TURP are about 3 percent.

Transurethral resection, as with open prostatectomies, can result in temporary or permanent impotence. There is no solid statistical data on the percentage of patients who become impotent after a TURP, although some figures suggest the number could be as high as one in five. The problem with these estimates is that many men are already impotent before having a TURP, which causes an upward bias in reported cases. Impotence after prostate surgery is discussed at length in Chapter 7. Today, impotence can be effectively overcome with modern medical treatments, including penile implants.

In a majority of cases, men do experience retrograde ejaculation, when there is no semen discharge through the penis, resulting in an infertility problem for men who wish to father children. But this problem can also be overcome, as you will see in Chapter 8.

While temporary incontinence is common after a TURP, long-term incontinence is no more than a 1.5-percent possibility. Incontinence and its treatment is discussed in Chapter 8.

Depending on where you live and assuming you have no complications, the total cost of a TURP could be in the $10,000 to $15,000 range (based on typical

1998 fees). There are usually few problems today regarding insurance coverage. However, TURP is one of the most common operations paid for by Medicare and, given the deepening health care crisis, Medicare and private carriers will probably try to limit this coverage. Their most likely argument will be over the point at which BPH ceases to be tolerable or safe for a given patient. One important tip for men who need BPH surgery—even should there be no doubt about your need for it—be sure your urologist gets written pre-operative approval from your insurance carrier and, when indicated, a second opinion, too.

Some Promising New Surgical Procedures

There has probably been more research conducted into prostate enlargement treatment during the past two decades than during the history of urology. Following are some of the new surgical procedures that may in time replace traditional transurethral resection and open prostatectomies in some patients.

Transurethral Incision of the Prostate (TUIP)

TUIP is a closed surgical procedure in which one or more small cuts are made inside the urethral channel in the area where the urethra passes through the prostate. The cut (or cuts) extends as far as the neck of the bladder. No enlarged prostate tissue is removed in a TUIP, but the procedure can result in improved urine flow.

TUIP's principal advantages are that it takes much less time to perform than conventional transurethral resections, is less expensive, and is easier on the patient than a TURP. Two other important advantages: There is considerably less chance of both postoperative impotence and retrograde ejaculation. The TUIP's principal disadvantages are that it is not suitable for patients with advanced prostate enlargement, and it may not result in a permanent cure. In contrast to a TURP, the procedure does not provide the urologist with a tissue sample for cancer biopsy. Given the importance of early cancer detection, a separate procedure is usually performed to obtain a biopsy sample when a TUIP is performed.

The TUIP made its initial appearance in the late seventies but is still not widely used. Typically, it is performed on men with unacceptable voiding difficulties, exhibiting relatively minor prostate enlargement. An especially appropriate candidate for TUIP would be a younger man with a voiding problem who wishes to avoid retrograde ejaculation because he wants to father children. When compared with a

TURP, a TUIP results in slightly less improvement of urine flow. Both procedures have about the same rate of re-operation, between 1 and 2 percent a year.

Transurethral Ultrasound-Guided Laser Prostatectomy (TULIP)

TULIP is an innovative closed surgical procedure employing ultrasound and laser technologies. The procedure first appeared in the late eighties and is still experimental.

In a TULIP, ultrasound and laser elements within a balloon are inserted into the urethra and the balloon is inflated. The urologist then removes excess prostate tissue using the laser. The ultrasound element provides an image the urologist uses to guide the cutting laser. This method is so precise that the beam delivers a cutting spot only 2.8mm in diameter, a bit more than a tenth of an inch wide.

TULIP offers a number of important advantages compared with conventional transurethral resection, chief among them is the possibility of using only local anesthesia. That can be important to patients who may have adverse or even life-threatening reactions to general anesthesia. The procedure usually takes only a few minutes and in some cases can be performed as an outpatient. Because of the precise cutting, there is also considerably less blood loss, faster postoperative healing, and lessened possibility of side effects, especially incontinence.

TULIP's disadvantages include greater expense and a shortage of urologists suitably trained to perform it. The cost should come down in the future as briefer periods of time in the hospital and the operating room balance out the significantly higher cost of the laser equipment. The availability of urologists who can perform the procedure can be expected to solve itself in time. A final disadvantage is that a TULIP, similar to a transurethral incision of the prostate, produces no tissue for cancer biopsy, thus necessitating a separate procedure.

Trans-Urethral Needle Ablation (TUNA)

Radio frequency energy is also being used to treat BPH, with clinical trials underway of this new technique. TUNA involves insertion of tiny needles into the prostate via a special catheter. The needles carry radio waves which riddle the prostate with little holes to loosen the tissue's hold on the urethra. Early results are promising, and, if approved, the procedure may be inexpensive since it works off a battery-operated device.

What You Need to Know About Prostatectomy

Although many of the recent, more notable advances in treating enlarged prostates are already becoming part of everyday urology practice, prostatectomy is likely to remain the treatment for many men for some time. Here are answers to some of the most frequently asked questions by men who are facing some type of prostatectomy:

QUESTION: How dangerous is the operation?

ANSWER: Every surgical procedure, even removing a skin blemish, involves some risk. In transurethral resectomy, the risk is a scant seven-tenths of a percent (0.7 percent). As a comparison, your chances of dying from the Whipple operation for pancreatic cancer is about 10 percent. Be assured that if you are generally healthy—not obese, with good cardiovascular fitness and without complicating problems such as diabetes—your chances of dying from a prostatectomy are even less than the seven-tenths norm.

QUESTION: Will the operation and postoperative recovery be very painful?

ANSWER: No to both. Understandably, most men are concerned about having a resectoscope inserted into their penises during a TURP, but their fear is a lot worse than the reality. A tranquilizer before the operation will help you overcome your apprehension and appropriate local anesthesia will take care of the rest. And under anesthesia, you will experience no pain during an open prostatectomy.

In TURPs, there is normally little if any postoperative pain, but after an open prostatectomy, you will usually notice some tenderness at the site of the abdominal incision. With pain-relieving medication, your discomfort can be kept minimal. Many men worry about the catheter inserted into their penises following both TURPs and open prostatectomies. Catheters sometimes cause bladder spasms, but that is controllable with medication.

QUESTION: What about my future sex life? Will I still be able to father children?

ANSWER: The first question is asked by almost all my patients, the second, not as often, because most men who need prostatectomies are already at an age and in a family situation where fathering children is no longer a concern. However, as we've seen, both impotence and retrograde ejaculation are sometimes consequences of a prostatectomy. The odds are you won't develop impotence, but even if you do, it doesn't mean the end of your sex life. Effective treatments are discussed in Chapter 7. In fact, your sex life may improve once the physical and emotional burden of voiding difficulties is lifted. You will probably experience retrograde ejaculation after a prostatectomy, but it should not adversely affect your sex life. As Chapter 8 points out, it might make fathering children more complicated, but not impossible.

QUESTION: Is it true many men experience serious incontinence and pass blood in their urine following a prostatectomy?

ANSWER: You will likely have some difficulty controlling your urine flow after a prostatectomy, but the problem usually ends in a few weeks. As mentioned previously, your odds of avoiding a long-term incontinence problem are quite good. Besides temporary incontinence after the operation, you will probably experience some mild discomfort when urinating. That, too, should clear up shortly.

You can expect to see some blood in your urine, which can be quite unsettling, because many men fear bleeding from the penis. Finding blood in your urine after a prostatectomy is normal and is nothing to be concerned about unless it continues beyond the normal recovery period (see below). You can help yourself by drinking plenty of liquids during your recovery.

QUESTION: Can there be any other complications?

ANSWER: Other complications are rare. One that might arise from a TURP would be discovery of large stones or pouches in the bladder. In those cases, your urologist may decide to terminate the TURP and perform an open prostatectomy so he can treat the bladder problems as well as your prostate enlargement. In that event, you'll have a longer hospital stay than you expected, but you'll avoid future difficulties.

Postoperative bladder or prostate infections and sepsis (blood poisoning) are also possible. Suitable medications will prevent such infections and treat them, if need be. To avoid infections, urologists routinely check for prostatitis before they schedule a prostatectomy. Unless there is an emergency, the operation will not be performed until the prostatitis infection is cured.

QUESTION: How soon will I be back to normal?

ANSWER: Complete healing following either a TURP or an open prostatectomy can take up to six weeks. As discussed, laser surgery offers even more rapid healing. An extended recovery period does not mean you won't be able to go home and resume most of your normal activities, including going back to work, even if your job involves travel. Mild exercise, in particular walking, should be no problem and will in fact prove beneficial. With open prostatectomies, however, it is best to avoid heavy physical activity and automobile driving until your abdominal incision is fully healed.

QUESTION: Will I be fully cured and might the operation have to be repeated eventually?

ANSWER: Small boys often compete to see who can urinate the longest distance. Don't expect a prostatectomy to allow you to relive that and some of the other wonderful feats of childhood. But most men do achieve welcome and worthwhile relief following treatment, including a less frequent need to urinate, the ability to sleep though the night, reduced urinary hesitancy, and the end of urinary retention and urgency. As noted, the chances are few that a resumption of a benign growth inside your prostate will ever lead to a second operation.

Some Promising New Nonsurgical Procedures for Treating BPH

Recently, several innovative nonsurgical treatments for BPH have appeared. The most important are balloon dilatation, transurethral hyperthermia, and the use of urethral prostheses. These treatments are not considered surgery because none involve actual tissue cutting. They are, however, all invasive in nature as they require physical entry through the penis of medical devices designed to treat the enlargement.

Balloon Dilatation

Balloon dilatation, also known as balloon urethroplasty, is a new treatment first applied in the late eighties. The procedure does not yet have full FDA approval, although it is available experimentally in most major U.S. urban areas. Balloon dilatation to alleviate BPH owes much to previous work in cardiology, in particular to balloon angioplasty, a method for opening clogged arteries in the heart.

To treat BPH, a dilatation catheter incorporating an inflatable balloon is inserted into the penis and slipped through the previously lubricated urethra until the forward section of it passes through the prostate and enters the bladder. At that point, the balloon is roughly positioned in the area where excess prostate tissue is pinching the urethra. A fine adjustment of the balloon's position is made with a positioning control. Then the balloon is inflated to a high pressure, by injecting into it a stream of salt water. After it widens the urethral channel sufficiently, the balloon is deflated and the catheter is withdrawn.

The main advantage of balloon dilatation is avoiding surgery, with its consequent complications, either on a short- or long-term basis. Jason, my basketball coach patient, opted for balloon dilatation hoping to postpone surgery long enough for the new drugs being developed to treat BPH to become generally available and be proved effective. Other advantages: Balloon dilatation generally takes only about a half hour, requires only local anesthesia, can be performed as an outpatient, and its side effects are rare. Although experimental, the procedure should be covered by your insurance, although it is best to check in advance.

The principal disadvantages of balloon dilatation: It does not work on many patients and does not necessarily provide a permanent cure. While there *is* some improvement in as many as nine out of every ten men, significant relief of voiding difficulties is reported by only about one in five men with severe prostate enlargement. When men have moderate enlargement or less, that figure rises to three in five. It is too soon to know how long the benefits will persist in typical patients. However, balloon dilatation can be repeated and may be worth a try, especially in cases with only moderate gland enlargement.

Transurethral Hyperthermia (TH)

Transurethral hyperthermia is an experimental procedure introduced in the late eighties. FDA-approved field trials are underway in several major U.S. cities and studies are also being conducted overseas. This procedure uses heat produced by microwave radiation to treat a urinary obstruction.

In general principle, hyperthermia is roughly similar to "sweat box" techniques used many years ago, only very tightly targeted to the prostate and done with either microwaves or electrodes. Through a probe inserted into the urethra, and a device called a Prostatron positioned in the rectum, microwave treatment basically burns a new channel through the muscular and glandular tissue. The prostate can remain irritated until the tissue dies and is sloughed off by the body. A typical course of therapy involves ten treatments of about one hour which do not require a hospital stay. Hyperthermia is being used to treat BPH and prostate cancer, although temperatures used in BPH treatment are slightly higher than those used to treat prostate cancer.

The principal advantages of transurethral hyperthermia: It is easy to tolerate, requires only local anesthesia, and can be performed in a urologist's office as an outpatient. The treatment sessions are brief and, to date, the results indicate the possibility of significant improvement of a BPH condition after only one or two sessions.

Urethral Stents

A mechanical device, a urethral stent is inserted into the urethra to keep open the urinary channel. At this time, these devices are at an early stage of development. Most now undergoing study are spiral wires that apply outward pressure on the urethral wall and keep the channel open. Typically, the devices are fabricated from corrosion-resistant metal such as stainless steel.

The main advantage of a urethral prosthesis is avoiding surgery, particularly important for older men in poor health who are poor surgical risks. Their disadvantages include medical lack of knowledge of the long-term effect of implanting these devices, possibly including incontinence. There is also some possibility of infection. Consequently, urethral prostheses are mostly limited to older patients.

Both temporary and permanent stents are being developed. Temporary stents are simple and inexpensive, but they need to be replaced. Permanent stents last longer, and are constructed of a material which actually receives an inner coating of new cells which makes it more like a part of the body.

Symptoms such as incontinence or the retention of urine can sometimes be resolved by a very slight repositioning of the stent.

In general, stents are most effective when the problem is limited to a stricture (contraction) of the urethra itself. With BPH, continued growth (including into the spirals of the stent) can negate the effect of the device.

What about Drugs?

The patient is rare who does not prefer taking a drug that is safe and effective, reasonably priced, and has minimal side effects to undergoing surgery. Given the growing potential of the BPH market, major drug manufacturers have been scrambling to develop products that will do the job.

However, the poorly understood association between prostate enlargement and high cholesterol levels has led to some prior use of cholesterol-lowering agents in treating BPH. Some of the drugs used principally to treat fungus infections, candicidin and amphotericin B, have lowered cholesterol levels in the prostate. These cholesterol-lowering drugs also provide positive benefits with respect to heart attack and stroke, as well as prostate enlargement.

There is more interest currently in two other types of drugs. The first are alpha adrenergic blockers, believed to work because they help relax the smooth muscles of the prostate and allow improved urine flow through the urethra. The second are drugs that interfere with the normal action of testosterone within the prostate.

Alpha Adrenergic Blockers

Alpha adrenergic blockers are mainly used to treat high blood pressure. However, clinical trials have shown that four alpha blockers—phenoxybenzamine, prazosin, doxasozin, and terazosin—also help patients with enlarged prostates. The equivalent success rate with these medications is about 70 percent. These drugs seem to work by interfering with certain receptor sites in the smooth muscles of enlarged prostate tissues and in the prostate capsule that surrounds the gland. When that occurs, pressure on the urethra is relieved and better voiding can be the result.

Of these three drugs, terazosin, sold under the name Hytrin, has received the most attention. Its manufacturer, Abbott Laboratories, filed for FDA approval to promote Hytrin as a BPH treatment. However, some urologists are already prescribing the drug because, under FDA rules, a drug on the market that has been approved for one use, in this case hypertension, can legally be prescribed by a physician for other conditions. But except for research purposes, a manufacturer cannot promote alternate use without FDA approval.

Hytrin's principal advantage is that, in about two-thirds of all patients, it results in speedy symptomatic relief and thus may help avoid surgery. The drug also appears to be suitable for once-a-day dosage. One disadvantage is that the drug does not halt tumor growth and therefore it is no cure for BPH. Hytrin also has side effects, including episodes of dizziness, fatigue, and fainting. While not usually too serious, they are symptoms of abnormally low blood pressure, suggesting the drug may not be suitable for patients who, in the absence of any medication, regularly exhibit abnormally low blood pressure readings. For men with high blood pressure, these side effects do not generally present a problem.

Drugs That Control Testosterone

Drugs controlling or countering testosterone effects have been receiving considerable attention recently and are therefore discussed at greater length here. Historically, the earliest drugs treating enlarged prostates were antitestosterone agents, including estrogen, the female hormone. Drugs of that nature were often found to be effective in reducing prostate size. However, they do lower testosterone levels throughout the body, not only in the prostate. Unfortunately, their side effects in other parts of the body were too often similar to castration—impotence, lost or markedly lower libido, loss of body vigor, and the appearance of feminine physical characteristics, including enlarged breasts.

Some newer drugs at advanced stages of development also work by interacting with testosterone, but their effects are generally restricted to the prostate. One reason for some of the newer drugs to be more selective is that just as there is "good" and "bad" cholesterol, there is also "good" and "bad" testosterone. Good testosterone is manufactured in the testicles, where the level of production is governed by enzymes produced in the important hypothalamus and pituitary glands. Bad testosterone, or dihydrotestosterone (DHT), is produced inside the prostate from good testosterone supplied from the testicles. DHT is needed for normal physical development at puberty, but later in life it actually causes excess prostate tissue growth. The newer drugs are designed to counter DHT inside the prostate, without preventing the good testosterone from doing its vital work in other parts of the body.

One promising drug for controlling bad testosterone is flutamide, sold under the name Eulexin. Flutamide is also used to treat prostate cancer and seems to work by binding rapidly to certain sites in the prostate. This action effectively blocks DHT, which must also bind to the same sites before it can cause prostate tissue growth.

Flutamide appears to be effective in many patients. Side effects are not generally severe, but may include hot flashes, libido loss, impotence, and gastrointestinal problems. The drug is undergoing clinical trials and has yet to receive FDA approval for general distribution.

Most current interest is centered on a drug whose trade name is Proscar from the large pharmaceutical manufacturer Merck & Co. The exciting potential for this drug has attracted not only urologists, but the Wall Street investment community. Proscar interferes with 5-alpha reductase, an enzyme found inside the prostate. When it does, the conversion of good testosterone into the bad DHT cannot occur.

An oral dose of 5 mg per day results in a 75 percent decrease in serum DHT levels. The equivalent success rate seems to be about 70 percent, but the drug must be taken indefinitely to thwart a return of the symptoms.

How the Merck scientists got the idea for Proscar is worth relating. In a mountain village on a small Caribbean island, a group of unfortunate men suffered from a form of hermaphroditism. Because at birth the sexual organs of these men appeared to be female, the children were raised as girls. At puberty, however, the group suddenly began to grow noticeable male sexual organs, plus exhibit other masculine features, such as beards and deep voices. There was one notable exception; their prostates continued to remain small. Research at Cornell Medical College determined that all these men suffered from a genetic defect that caused a deficiency in a critical enzyme, 5-alpha reductase. When Merck learned of that, the race was to produce a drug that would counter the enzyme; the reasoning, correct as it turned out, was that this would result in lower levels of DHT in the prostate.

Field studies conducted by Merck suggest that more than half of all men who take a tablet of Proscar each day for six months will experience better voiding and even more will have fewer episodes of urgency. But the drug is no panacea. Proscar must be taken for about six months before there is significant shrinking of the prostate and about 3.5 percent of users experience impotence. Impotence disappears when the drug is discontinued. Proscar has mostly been tested with older men, so its suitability in younger patients has yet to be determined.

During 1992, the FDA approved Proscar for general distribution. There is little doubt that the drug will be an important tool for future BPH treatment. There is some concern that if the drug is widely prescribed by physicians other than urologists, many men will fail to have their prostate conditions monitored adequately. A special problem is that patients who take Proscar may in some instances exhibit false readings when taking the PSA test for prostate cancer. This points up the vital importance of frequent digital rectal examinations by an experienced urologist.

Finisteride works on men whose BPH is primarily glandular rather than muscular, therefore making it more susceptible to hormonal manipulations. In one study of 1,600 men, finisteride shrank prostate size by an average of 25 percent over a two-year period. However, some evidence exists that finisteride actually assists the growth of prostate cancer in a small percentage of men who use it, mostly men who are at higher risk because of their age, race, or family history of prostate cancer. These men might be advised not to take finisteride, and to seek other types of treatments for BPH.

Since finisteride is quite new, several questions remain unanswered. A research study due to be completed in the year 2000 is underway at the National Cancer Institute to test the viability of using finisteride as a chemopreventative agent for BPH or prostate cancer. This study will track 18,000 men who began the trial with PSA test results below 3 ng/ml over a number of years.

So, your chances of avoiding significant prostate enlargement at some point in your life are not good. But if you are lucky, your condition may never need aggressive treatment or, in particular, surgery. Never delay treatment, however, if there is any danger of bladder damage or there's a serious deterioration in your quality of life.

Transurethral resection has become the most common treatment for enlarged prostates and will probably remain so for the immediate future. This surgical procedure is safe and effective in almost all men and its side effects are minimal or treatable. A number of exciting surgical and nonsurgical procedures, along with promising new drugs, are appearing and will promise genuine hope to men in years to come.

CHAPTER 6

Prostate Cancer:
There Is Good News

The previous chapter covered the fairly common problem of benign prostate enlargement. This chapter deals with prostate tumors that are found not to be benign and instead are malignant or cancerous.

Benign prostatic hyperplasia (BPH) and prostate cancer have some factors in common. These diseases are characterized by excessive growth of prostate tissue, and with each disease, testosterone is an important factor that stimulates this growth. They are typically diseases of older men, although prostate cancer more usually strikes quite late in life. However, there is one important difference: In BPH, excess tissue growth is confined to the inside of the prostate and adverse consequences of this growth are limited to its impact on the adjacent urinary system. But prostate cancer can escape the confines of the prostate and spread to other parts of the body, with potentially serious, if not fatal, consequences.

Prostate cancer is treatable and the chances of success are especially favorable when the disease is detected early. This chapter will provide important information on the disease and should help you put the problem of prostate cancer and its treatment into proper perspective. You will also learn how the disease progresses in stages, what the currently available treatment tools are, and which treatment methods are most appropriate at each stage. Promising treatment approaches are now being studied that offer great hope to any man with prostate cancer.

Putting Prostate Cancer in Proper Perspective

One of the worst tasks any physician faces is telling patients they have cancer. Cliff, a fifty-year-old building contractor, took it very hard when I had to tell him he had prostate cancer. He refused to listen to anything I said about the recommended treatment and his excellent prognosis for recovery and he immediately rushed out of my office.

For more than a week, I didn't hear from Cliff and was about to call him to urge prompt treatment. Fortunately, he telephoned me first. Several hours later in my office, Cliff, an avid yachtsman, told me he had spent the week sailing alone along the Gulf Coast in his thirty-five-foot sloop. For a while, he had considered pointing the bow of his boat south and just sailing away.

While Cliff's instant reaction to learning he had prostate cancer was extreme, it wasn't unusual. Despite all the remarkable advances in medical science, mentioning the dreaded "C word" (cancer) still evokes strong emotions. Shock, denial, and resignation are common emotional responses from new cancer patients. Unfortunately, too many of us still believe cancer is an automatic death sentence.

Its emotional impact and the many erroneous beliefs about cancer add to the initial burden of cancer patients. Patients often report being overwhelmed by the gush of concern and sympathy from family members. Other patients still report that longtime friends and fellow employees avoid them, in the mistaken belief that the disease is contagious. Cancer patients, despite otherwise good health and with excellent future prospects, often have great difficulty getting a job or health and life insurance coverage. There has been some discussion that the recently enacted federal Americans with Disabilities Act may be amended to include discrimination against cancer patients.

So don't be taken in by rumors and myths, and don't be discouraged. Physicians often remark that patients forearmed with the truth about cancer and who have a generally positive attitude demonstrate the best prospects for successful recovery. There is really no objective proof that cancer survival is related to a patient's emotional state, but it is reasonable to believe that informed patients are quicker to seek help and benefit from their spirit of cooperation during treatment.

Cliff's case is instructive. After overcoming his initial shock and learning the truth about his situation, he became a perfect patient. His cancer was detected early, so the complete surgical removal of his prostate by radical prostatectomy was fully effective. Since then, Cliff has experienced six happy and productive years and there has been no sign of recurrent malignancy. He feels great and continues to enjoy a fully satisfying sex life. Cliff still tries to apologize for his initial panic when I told him he had prostate cancer.

Cancer: When Cells Get out of Control

Cancer is actually a family of diseases in which something goes wrong in the DNA, the chemical code programmed into every living cell. When cancer is present, affected cells multiply rapidly. Depending on the type of cancer, a malignant tumor known medically as a carcinoma may form at the original disease site. Contrary to common belief, cancer cells are not cannibals that feed on nearby healthy cells. Instead, the body is damaged when the growing mass of carcinoma eventually interferes adversely with the normal function of nearby tissue.

If local damage were all that resulted, that would be bad enough, but at least the damage would be restricted. However, cancerous cells can metastasize or spread from their original site to other parts of the body. "Cancer" means crab in Latin. In naming the disease, the ancients drew an analogy between the outreaching persistent claws of the crab and the spread of cancer throughout the body.

The triggers for uncontrolled cell growth are not fully understood. Every cell in your body is subject to continuing mutation, a form of chemical change in the DNA code that governs cell function, including reproduction. Each day an average body cell experiences more than 5,000 individual mutations triggered by some external force. Most cell mutations are harmless, but if the mechanism controlling reproduction in even a single cell is affected adversely, cancerous growth can result.

The external force triggering dangerous mutations in some cancers has been attributed to viruses. Other cancers have been linked to substances known as carcinogens—hazardous chemicals in food, polluted air, or elsewhere in the environment, as well as exposure to radioactivity, heat, and intense sunlight.

One of the most exciting recent developments was the discovery in 1989 of the "guardian" p53 gene. Present in every cell, p53 is believed to play a key role in tumor suppression, possibly explaining why so few of the 5,000 daily mutations in each of the enormous number of cells in your body actually result in cancer. Still inconclusive evidence suggests cancer will appear when some damage occurs to the p53 itself. In such circumstances, the gene may be damaged so that its action actually serves to *promote* cancer. If these preliminary findings are valid, science may be closer to unraveling a basic mystery of cancer, bringing with it the possibility of more effective cures and even a means of preventing cancer.

Some Facts About Prostate Cancer

Prostate cancer is characterized by the growth within the gland of a malignant tumor, medically known as an "adenocarcinoma." This tumor is defined as a "primary cancer" because its growth is triggered by an event within the prostate, not by the invasion of cancerous cells from some other part of the body. Most often, growth of an adenocarcinoma occurs first in the outer rear region of the prostate. As growth continues, the tumor may spread deep into the interior of the gland. In time, the malignancy may establish footholds in the various organs surrounding the prostate, eventually spreading to many other parts of the body. Such adenocarcinomas arising in the glandular units or *acini* comprise some 95 percent of all prostate cancers. The small remaining percentage of prostate cancers are other types—a few resemble bladder cancers, and a few begin in the muscles or the excretory ducts of the prostate gland.

In 1995, the American Cancer Society estimated that approximately 200,000 men would be diagnosed with prostate cancer. As the population is aging, instances of prostate cancer are increasing.

What Are The Symptoms of Prostate Cancer?

Unfortunately, most of the time, cancer which is confined to the prostate gland has no symptoms at all. All of the symptoms may be attributed to BPH, or to other causes such as the aging process. This is the reason many men don't realize they have a problem until the cancer has spread beyond the prostate—which is when between 25 to 35 percent of cases are discovered.

The first noticeable symptom is often *induration* or hardening of the prostate gland. This is what a urologist can discover with a DRE, which allows some prostate cancers to be detected in its early stages. Beyond that, another symptom of prostate cancer is an impeded flow of urine from the bladder, resulting in painful urination, slowing of the stream, difficulty starting to urinate, dribbling, incomplete bladder emptying, increased frequency of urination, or increased urination at night—also symptoms which may be mistaken for BPH. If cancer has spread to other organs, symptoms may show up in those areas—such as shortness of breath for lung metastases, or hip or lower back pain for metastasis to the bone.

What Causes Prostate Cancer?

Patients often ask me what caused their prostate cancer. Unfortunately, there is no definitive answer, not too surprising since, despite recent advances in medical science, a specific cause cannot be identified in more than half of all cancer types. In cases where a cause has been located scientifically, smoking is the most frequent culprit.

In prostate cancer, there is some evidence that a diet high in fat may increase the odds. However, no link has yet been found between prostate cancer and anything else you personally control, such as alcohol, tobacco, or other drugs. There is some evidence that men exposed in the workplace to cadmium, a fairly toxic metallic element, are at slightly greater risk. Cadmium is present in storage battery manufacture, metal alloys, and electroplating. Men working in these industries should be careful to follow safety rules, and to have periodic prostate examinations.

Genetics may be a factor, too, as revealed by statistics that suggest men with a father or brother who had prostate cancer have a considerably higher risk for the disease. Black Americans have the highest known incidence of prostate cancer in the world. New cases are reported in African Americans at a rate per 100,000, almost double that of Caucasians. Genetics might also be a factor, but so could environmental conditions or even a combination of the two.

First degree relatives who are considered can be either on the father's or the mother's side. Genetically, the highest risk group are men who have had both first and second degree relatives with prostate cancer. Men in these high-risk groups are also more likely to get prostate cancer at a younger age, and are therefore advised to get a DRE and PSA test every year after they turn forty.

Hormones play a significant role. Testosterone stimulates malignant cell growth in the prostate. Prostate cancer is rare in men who were castrated before the usual onset age for the disease. As we've seen, testosterone has the same effect in stimulating benign prostate enlargement. However, there is no evidence of any other connection between prostate cancer and BPH.

Early in 1993, two studies were reported in the *Journal of the American Medical Association* suggesting that men who had had vasectomies as long as twenty or so years ago have shown an increased incidence of prostate cancer. However, these studies are at odds with two earlier investigations indicating no such relationship. If you have had a vasectomy, don't panic. No study has yet demonstrated without qualification any increased risk of death from prostate cancer in vasectomized men. Earlier concerns about a possible relationship between vasectomy and cardiovascular disease were never substantiated either. Even so, taking the recent studies into account, the American Urological Association recommends that all men who had vasectomies more than twenty years ago or who were more than forty at the time of a vasectomy should have an annual digital rectal examination and the PSA test. I recommend the same plan to any patient whose close family relatives have a prostate cancer history. The American Urological Association is NOT recommending against vasectomy.

Finally, some studies suggest a possible relationship between prostate cancer and sexual behavior. A study at the University of Illinois suggested that a pattern of lifelong sexual repression was linked to increased incidence of prostate cancer, theorizing that a buildup of male hormones in the prostate might be the cause. While the link between prostate cancer and a lack of sex is not yet fully proved, as discussed in Chapter 4, there *is* a known connection between sexual abstinence and some prostate problems.

Who Gets Prostate Cancer?

Prostate cancer strikes men in all walks of life. Some recent cases have included Senator Robert Dole, the senate minority leader; Stan Musial, the great St. Louis Cardinals slugger; General Norman Schwarzkopf, hero of the Gulf War; Jerry Lewis, the entertainer; and Michael Milken, financier and convicted felon.

What Are My Chances?

At this time, new prostate cancer cases are diagnosed among American males in excess of 130,000 cases a year and that total is rising. After skin cancer, prostate cancer is the most common cancer among men in the United States. It is well ahead of the third most common type, lung cancer, which has about 100,000 new cases a year.

Based on these statistics, your chances as an American male of developing prostate cancer are about one in eleven, about the same rate as for women who develop breast cancer. There is no hard evidence but there is good reason to suspect that prostate cancer is actually more common in men than breast cancer is in women. Breast cancer has received extensive coverage by the media, and women have been strongly encouraged to undergo annual mammographies. Prostate cancer and the need for the digital rectal examination have not received nearly as much attention. Consequently, many cases of prostate cancer may be undiagnosed.

Your chances of getting prostate cancer increase significantly with age. In men under fifty, the disease is rare. However, the number of cases in younger men may increase chiefly because of improved diagnoses. As many as 30 percent of all men above fifty harbor some cancerous cells in the prostate, but only 1 percent of these men will develop cancer itself. About 80 percent of all prostate cancer cases are diagnosed in men sixty-five and older. Cancerous cells are detected in the prostate in most men in their eighties, although octogenarians usually die from heart disease, pneumonia, and other disorders of old age, not from prostate cancer.

The American Cancer Society predicted about 34,000 American men would die from prostate cancer in 1998. That is about a third of the rate for men who die from lung cancer, but ahead of the colon and rectal cancer death rates. The total deaths annually from prostate cancer has been increasing, mainly because of a growing population of older American men. Because of their age, they are at increased risk for prostate cancer, not from any failure of medicine or the presence of anything new in the environment.

Your overall chances with prostate cancer are dependent on how far the disease has progressed when it is first diagnosed. The earlier the detection, the easier and more effective the treatment.

Prostate Cancer: Disease in Four Stages

Typically, prostate cancer progresses in four distinct stages, known to urologists as A, B, C, and D (see Figure 6.1). Tests indicate the physical volume of the malignancy and how far it has spread from its initial site of origin within the prostate capsule, which determines the "stage" (sometimes called the "staging") of the disease.

The tests that determine the stage of prostate cancer were discussed in Chapter 2. The most important are the digital rectal examination, tissue biopsy, blood chemistry analysis, prostate specific antigen (PSA), prostatic acid phosphatase (PAP), transrectal ultrasound, bone scan, chest X-ray, magnetic resonance imaging (MRI), computerized tomography (CT), and intravenous pyelograms. These tests not only determine the progress of the disease at its first diagnosis, but are essential for determining the most effective treatment, and in monitoring the course of the disease during treatment.

Another test you may encounter during the staging process is the Gleason grading system, which is the most widely used and accepted of several grading systems. Prostate cancer is different from almost any other type of cancer in that it often contains a mixture of several types of aggressive and nonaggressive cancer cells. Aggressive, poorly-differentiated cancer cells can grow and spread much faster than passive well-differentiated cancer cells. The Gleason system ranks the two most populous groups of cancer cells on a scale of one to five, with one the best grade. These two scores are added together to produce a score between two and ten. Higher Gleason grading numbers indicate a more malignant tumor. As a word of caution, physicians are not in perfect agreement as to how they interpret the results of these and other grading tests. A urologist looks at all available test results to arrive at a determination of the four stages of prostate cancer.

Stage A—Tumor Confined to the Prostate, but Difficult to Detect

In Stage A prostate cancer, the malignant tumor is confined entirely within the capsule encasing the prostate. At this stage, the tumor may have been present for years without the patient's noticing symptoms. For that reason, the home tests discussed in Chapter 9 are not of much value, although you should promptly have a urologist investigate any evidence of blood in your urine and semen.

The tumor is so small in Stage A that it normally escapes detection during the digital rectal examination. Until recently, diagnoses of Stage A prostate cancer have been rare, and when they do occur, it is usually from biopsies performed routinely on tissue samples obtained during prostatectomies conducted to treat benign prostate enlargement. If a biopsy reveals evidence of cancer in no more than 5 percent of the tissue, the cancer is said to be in sub-Stage A_1. If it has progressed beyond 5 percent, the cancer is in sub-Stage A_2.

Given the importance of early diagnosis, it would be a major advance if all prostate cancers could be detected in Stage A_1. Fortunately, as discussed in Chapter 2, a new diagnostic tool is available: the prostate specific antigen, or PSA, test. This test can be performed simply and inexpensively on a patient's blood sample,

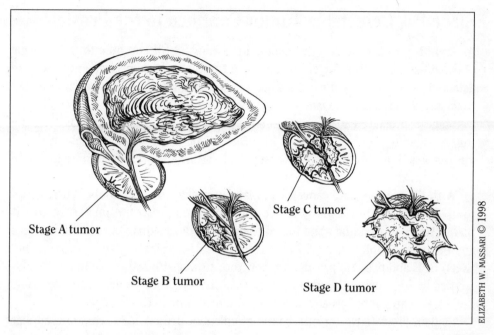

Stage A tumor

Stage B tumor

Stage C tumor

Stage D tumor

ELIZABETH W. MASSARI © 1998

Figure 6.1 *The Four Stages of Prostate Cancer*

and will detect Stage A prostate cancer in many cases. However, there is some concern among urologists with the PSA test, largely because it sometimes diagnoses cancer when it is not actually present (a false positive). And this test sometimes suggests the reverse (a false negative). Nevertheless, the American Urological Association recommends an annual PSA screening for men fifty and older. I think this is sensible.

The possibility of widespread use of Proscar for BPH treatment adds further complications. Because men who avoid prostatectomies by using Proscar are not subject to routine tissue biopsy, some early cases of prostate cancer may escape detection. Proscar use may also affect PSA results.

In the future, there is reason to believe the PSA test will be improved, detecting more cases of prostate cancer during Stage A. Newer diagnostic tools may also emerge, a good possibility being the DNA probes, highly advanced diagnostic systems offering the promise of easy detection of Stage A prostate cancer based on determining the genetic structure of substances found in urine or semen samples.

Stage B—Detectable Tumor Confined to the Prostate

In Stage B prostate cancer, the malignant tumor is still confined to the interior of the prostate. At this stage, however, the tumor has grown large enough to be detected by a urologist during a digital rectal examination. Most early prostate cancer is detected that way.

Stage B prostate cancer is also divided into two sub-stages. In Stage B_1, the tumor is found in only one lobe of the prostate and is less than 2cm (about three-fourths of an inch) in diameter. In Stage B_2, the tumor is present in more than one lobe or is greater than 2cm in size.

With Stage B prostate cancer, you may not notice any symptoms. When symptoms do appear, they usually affect voiding: frequent urination (especially at night), urgency, hesitancy, and intermittent or reduced urinary stream. If you have any of these symptoms, it will take a urological examination to distinguish between BPH and possible prostate cancer. Your urologist may be able to tell the difference by feel during the digital rectal examination. Your urologist will probably order a PSA and, if he has any further doubt, recommend tissue biopsy.

Stage B prostate cancer may be symptomless or demonstrate symptoms similar to BPH, which points up the importance of periodic urological examinations. It also suggests the importance of consulting your urologist if you observe these symptoms.

Stage C—When the Tumor Leaves the Prostate

Prostate cancer is in Stage C when the malignant tumor manages to escape the confines of the prostate capsule to invade adjacent body areas, especially the seminal vesicles. In Stage C, the tumor has usually become so large that it creates pressure on the urethra. When that happens, voiding problems like those mentioned in connection with Stage B usually become more apparent. At Stage C, a patient may also feel mild pain in the prostate area.

Unfortunately, many patients do not visit a urologist until Stage C, but even then, the disease may still be treatable. If you are in Stage C, your urologist should have little difficulty spotting a problem during his digital rectal examination. To determine just how far the tumor has spread from the prostate in Stage C, the urologist may conduct an ultrasound test, especially of the seminal vesicles and may prescribe the prostatic acid phosphatase (PAP) test, which measures in the blood an abnormal rise of an enzyme produced in the prostate. The urologist may also order tissue biopsies of suspected areas outside the prostate.

Stage D—When the Tumor Spreads Throughout the Body

By Stage D of prostate cancer, the original tumor has metastasized or spread to other parts of the body. Common points of attack in Stage D are lymph nodes, bones, lungs, and liver. Eventually, other parts of the body may become involved. Stage D is sub-divided into Stages D_1 and D_2. In D_1, the malignancy has progressed to lymph nodes in the pelvic area. When that happens, the malignancy can spread to more distant parts of the body through the lymphatic system. In D_2, the malignancy has in fact reached more distant parts of the body.

Stage D patients usually experience very obvious voiding difficulties, serious fatigue, general malaise, and significant weight loss. They often have pain in their bones, especially in their upper thighs, lower back, and pelvic region.

During Stage D, chest X rays, computerized tomography, and magnetic resonance imaging determine the progress of the disease and identify those areas invaded by cancer. Any suspected areas are typically subjected to tissue biopsy. Bone scans employing radioisotopes that enhance X-ray images determine if there is bone involvement. The PAP, with other blood tests, may be used to determine if the disease has involved the liver or the bone marrow. An intravenous pyelogram may be ordered to determine if there has been any involvement in the kidney or bladder.

Treating Prostate Cancer

This section describes various methods for treating prostate cancer, regardless of its stage. You'll be told about treatments most often used at each of the four stages. In general, these cancer treatments are accepted by the American medical community or are now undergoing scientific investigation:

- Surgery
- Radiation therapy
- Drugs
- Hyperthermia
- Immunotherapy
- Gene therapy
- Watchful waiting

As with most cancers, prostate cancer treatment has been limited mainly to the first three approaches above—surgery, radiation therapy, and drugs (chemotherapy). Prostate cancer treatment programs commonly employ a combination of one or more of these three. Hyperthermia, immunotherapy, and gene therapy are still experimental, but may prove valuable in treating prostate and other cancers. Watchful waiting may be useful in certain situations. Chapter 11 discusses alternative treatments for prostate cancer that have yet to be accepted by the medical community.

Prostate Cancer Surgery

Prostate surgery involves cutting out the cancerous tissue with a scalpel or, more recently, a laser. Completely removing cancerous tissue eliminates the source of an existing malignancy, although it is possible that a new malignancy could develop on its own in the remaining healthy tissue. Implicit in surgery is possible surgical damage to healthy tissue and that the surgery may not remove entirely all the cancerous cells.

Castration—removing the testicles—is sometimes necessary in prostate cancer treatment. It is a surgical procedure whose object is to reduce testosterone production. Castration is discussed below in connection with drugs that treat prostate cancer.

To ensure complete removal of malignant tissue, thus eliminating the possibility of a new cancer developing on its own in healthy tissue, most urologists favor radical prostatectomy, removal of the entire prostate gland.

In Chapter 5, we described in connection with surgical treatment of benign prostate enlargement several ways to perform a prostatectomy. The first was perineal prostatectomy, where a cut is made through the area about halfway between the anus and the scrotum. The second was retropubic prostatectomy, a cut through the lower abdomen. The third was transurethral resection (TURP) by using an instrument inserted into the penis.

In a radical perineal prostatectomy for prostate cancer, the entire prostate gland is removed along with nearby tissues when there is any reason to suspect possible malignancy. This procedure offers the possibility of a permanent cure when the malignant tumor is sufficiently localized, but almost always causes impotence. Because a perineal prostatectomy is less physically affecting than a retropubic prostatectomy, it is sometimes used with older patients and those in poor health who may be higher surgical risks.

During the radical retropubic prostatectomy for prostate cancer, in order to provide additional reassurance, nearby pelvic lymph nodes are also removed. The operation is safe, although somewhat harder on a patient than perineal prostatectomy. Retropubic prostatectomy has some advantages over perineal prostatectomy as to impotence and incontinence. An additional factor favoring the retropubic procedure is that perineal prostatectomy is an older operation and younger urologists may lack training or experience in performing it.

With radical retropubic prostatectomy, there is a possibility of both impotence and incontinence. In the past several years, a new nerve-sparing surgical technique has been employed with retropubic prostatectomy that is said to reduce the possibility of impotence. This technique minimizes damage to the nerve bundle that controls erections. However, the effectiveness of this new procedure has not been well established. Regardless, as discussed in Chapter 8, treatments do exist for any impotence that follows radical prostatectomy. Fortunately, incontinence after a radical retropubic prostatectomy is found in only a few cases.

Sometimes, transurethral resection is used to remove cancerous prostate tissues. TURP does not remove the whole malignant tumor, so it does not provide a permanent cure. To some extent, it is used to provide relief from the voiding problems caused by prostate cancer, to obtain tissue samples for biopsy, and, as noted below, experimentally in association with laser surgery.

As we saw in Chapter 5, laser surgery is being used to treat benign prostate enlargement. Laser surgery is also being investigated experimentally for surgical treatment of prostate cancer. However, in connection with prostate cancer, it has attracted less attention than in BPH, owing to a prevailing belief among urologists that cancerous prostates should be removed entirely. That view tends to eliminate one of the major advantages of laser surgery, its highly accurate cutting. One approach now being considered is a combination of transurethral resection and laser surgery. In the first step of this technique, most of the prostate tissue is removed using a TURP. In the second step, all remaining prostate tissue is accurately removed with a laser beam guided by ultrasound imaging.

Cryosurgery and ultrasound surgery are both being investigated for prostate cancer treatment. Potentially, cryosurgery is easier on patients than conventional cutting. One advantage of cryoablation is that the patient experiences no bleeding or complications and can return home the day after the procedure. A major disadvantage is that it does not kill all the cancer cells on the first try. Therefore, this procedure may probably be best utilized on older men or as a salvage procedure after radiation therapy has failed. In ultrasound surgery, transrectal ultrasound, along with a computer in the procedure under study, first defines the tissue areas to be removed, then destroys malignant tissue with ultrasound bombardment. This technique also has the potential of making things easier on the patient.

A fascinating new technology, being investigated principally in the United Kingdom, uses robots in prostate surgery. In this emerging technique, a urologist programs the desired pattern of surgical cuts into a computer that controls a robot surgical device. The information is obtained from an earlier scan of the patient's internal anatomy. This technique extends the technology of navigation guidance systems that control cruise missile flight paths. Potentially, robot surgery offers more precise and deliberate cutting, and may make radical prostatectomies considerably easier on patients, reducing undesirable side effects, including impotence. Some medical observers think robot prostate surgery may be readily available before year 2000.

Radiation Therapy in Prostate Cancer Treatment

In radiation therapy, high-energy subatomic particles bombard and destroy prostate cancer cells. But radiation is inherently dangerous and always kills nearby healthy cells besides targeted cancerous cells. With a skilled radiologist, with lower levels of radiation, and with proper scheduling of treatment, "collateral" damage to healthy cells can be minimized. And when enough healthy cells manage to survive the radiation treatment, damaged healthy tissue can regenerate.

Radiation is scary to a general public conditioned by events such as the Chernobyl nuclear disaster in the Ukraine. However, there is no threat to life with the radiation levels used in standard medical practice.

Two methods are used to irradiate the prostate. In external-beam radiotherapy, the prostate is subjected to a brief period of bombardment by a focused beam of X-rays from an external machine. External-beam radiotherapy has been in general use for prostate cancer since the sixties. Radiation is applied as an outpatient, typically in a series of up to five-day-a-week sessions, usually conducted for about seven weeks. This treatment is absolutely painless.

A newer technique for irradiating the cancerous prostate began in the seventies and is gaining importance. Tiny capsules containing a radioactive substance are implanted surgically into the prostate tumor. This implantation is done under anesthesia with minimal discomfort. Known technically as interstitial radiation therapy, seed implantation generally uses Iodine 125 as its radioactive source. Once implanted, the seeds emit a continuous stream of radiation strong enough to kill cancerous cells for about one year. These seeds remain permanently; while there is always some continuing radiation, no harm or discomfort is caused to the patient.

There are side effects from both external-beam radiotherapy and seed implantation. In the former, about 25 percent of patients report symptoms including fatigue, nausea, diarrhea, frequent and painful urination, skin eruptions, and rectal bleeding or discomfort. In about all but 10 percent of patients, these symptoms usually disappear in less than three months. Drugs can help control some of these side effects. External-beam radiotherapy causes permanent impotence in from 20 to 40 percent of all patients.

Seed implantation, however, has considerably fewer and milder side effects, although some men do experience mild bladder or rectal irritations. Impotence and incontinence are reported at less than 10 percent and 5 percent, respectively, when Iodine 125 treatment is used. As will be discussed later, seed implantation is usually limited to early stages of prostate cancer.

In all radiation therapy, the possibility exists that some cancerous cells may not be destroyed. However, some studies have shown in about two out of three patients a disease-free, five-year survival rate with external-beam radiotherapy, and about the same for patients treated with seed implantation in combination with drugs. Generally, radiation therapy is a good choice for some men who prefer not to have surgery, or who, because of age or general physical condition, are not good surgery candidates.

A promising recent development is Palladium 103 seeds as a radioactive source, along with Iodine 125, sometimes also with X ray. Palladium treatment, which can be done as an outpatient, supported by ultrasound to guide the seed placement, appears to cause virtually no incontinence and a very low occurrence of impotence. Gus, a patient diagnosed with early prostate cancer, was playing golf two days after this procedure. He requested it after he learned that two friends who'd had radical prostatectomies have experienced impotence, and one became incontinent.

Prostate Cancer: Role of Drugs

Medical science has not yet developed a miracle drug that cures prostate cancer. Still, drugs do play an increasingly important and effective role in prostate cancer treatment. Drug therapy takes two forms: colon hormonal therapy and chemotherapy. The former, based on the pioneering work of Nobel Laureate Dr. Charles B. Huggins, has been used for about fifty years. The latter is still experimental.

Hormonal Therapy

Treatments for reducing testosterone production or blocking activity of this hormone can retard significantly the growth of prostate cancer in some patients, even reducing significantly the size of existing tumors in others. As is the case with benign prostate enlargement, it was recognized very early that castration would help men with prostate cancer. Although castration is surgery, it nevertheless represents a form of hormonal therapy.

Castration, or orchiectomy, involves the removal of the testicles and may even be performed as an outpatient with a local anesthetic. Neither the procedure itself nor recovery from it is painful. Contrary to common belief, removing the testicles does not always result in a loss of erections. As you will see in the following chapter, even in a castrated male, there are ways to deal with impotence.

Today, castration is rarely performed on men who have benign prostate enlargement, but it still has some role in prostate cancer treatment. It is widely employed in testicular cancer treatment. The continuing use of castration to treat prostate cancer is due principally to its obvious effectiveness in eliminating testosterone production, except for the small amount of the hormone produced in the adrenal glands. Within three hours of castration, testosterone levels drop by 95 percent, and they remain at that level, called the "castrate range." This is the standard against which hormonal drugs are judged.

Following orchiectomy, some men obtain silicone testicle implants for cosmetic purposes. These implants have aroused widespread public controversy in connection with silicone breast implants in women. Concern about the breast implants has arisen because of silicone leakage. But in testicle implants, liquid silicone is not used, so there have been few problems with them.

Of course, not all men opt for testicle implants, since there are few circumstances where the appearance of the genitals is of much concern. In others, though, the missing testicles raise psychological problems like those experienced by women after mastectomy.

Fortunately, today there are increasingly effective alternatives to castration. One possibility is the use of female hormones, including estrogen, to treat prostate cancer. However, this hormone causes undesirable side effects, as noted in Chapter 5. Another class of female hormones are the progestins which block the effect of androgens on prostate cancer. Megestrol (MGA or Megace) is one such hormone. These hormones don't have the risk of heart side effects, but they unfortunately stop working after about six to nine months. Therefore, there is increasing preference for "luteinizing hormone-releasing hormone" therapy, or LHRH.

Luteinizing hormone-releasing therapy involves a drug known as a LHRH analog. This substance chemically blocks the action of testosterone produced in the testicles. LHRH results are similar to castration and estrogen therapy, but with few of their inherent disadvantages.

Typically, patients treated with LHRH are injected about once a month at their urologist's office. Some men have experienced hot flashes, general pain and malaise, and gastrointestinal side effects. Most of these problems can be controlled with appropriate drugs, but impotence and libido loss are also possible. A number of LHRH analogs have been tested, but most current interest centers on a drug known as leuprolide, sold under the name Lupron.

LHRH therapy is often used in combination with antiandrogen therapy. Androgens are drugs that block the small additional amounts of testosterone produced in the adrenal glands. Flutamide, sold under the name Eulexin, has been one of the most frequently prescribed antiandrogens. As noted in Chapter 5, this drug is also used to treat BPH and has had certain side effects. Other antiandrogens that have shown promise include goserelin acetate, sold under the name Zoladex, and aminoglutithamide, sold as Cytraden. Bicalutamide (Casodex), an improved antiestrogen, was recently approved by the FDA—it may be used as an alternative to flutamide.

Other promising newer drugs with particular uses include ketoconazole, which suppresses testosterone production; liarozole, a hydroxylase/lyase inhibitor; and suramin, may well be a forerunner to a new class of drugs which act via growth factor antagonism, because it may work on hormone-resistant cells.

When LHRH and antiandrogen therapy are used in combination, side effects can include nausea, diarrhea, hot flashes, and vomiting. Impotence is also possible. Combination therapy, however, is often considerably more effective than LHRH therapy alone. This strategy is called an estrogen blockade, and it may one day become a standard treatment for some stages of prostate cancer. Some very promising work is being done using neoadjuvant hormone blockade therapy in an attempt to drive cancer which has escaped from the prostate capsule back into the capsule prior to surgery or radiation therapy. Neoadjuvant therapy occurs prior to the main therapy. It could be useful in treating prostate cancer if it destroys enough cancerous cells to change surgical margins from positive (cancerous) to negative (noncancerous), and if it cleans up residual microscopic metastases of cancer cells which may have spread to other sites such as the bone. Several studies indicate that hormone blockade does reduce the size of the prostate cancer, but these promising early results must be proven over the long term. If long-term results verify what proponents of this therapy believe, neoadjuvant hormone blockage therapy will become as common in treating prostate cancer as adjuvant therapy has become in treating breast cancer (and perhaps as successful). If this therapy lives up to its promise over the long term, men with later stage prostate cancers may experience the same low incidence of relapse as men whose prostate cancer is detected earlier.

The pace of hormonal therapy research has been accelerating, and new drugs are coming to my attention almost daily. One interesting drug reported to have possible value in treating prostate and other cancers is mifepristine, a drug developed in France, sold under the name RU-486. The drug is being sold for family planning purposes in several countries, but because RU-486 in effect induces abortion, its importation to the United States, even for research into other applications, has been severely restricted.

Although hormone therapy does not cure cancer, perhaps 80 to 85 percent of the men who receive hormonal therapy benefit somewhat—such as shrinkage of the tumor, relief of a urinary obstruction, lessened bone pain, increased appetite, mitigation of anemia, and reduced PSA levels. These effects stop when hormone therapy is stopped. How well hormone therapy works depends on the tumor itself—tumors with more hormone-sensitive cells will show a greater response. One study showed identical survival rates between patients who began hormone therapy immediately, and those who started it at a later time. In theory, hormone therapy could be used to prevent prostate cancer, but the side effects that many men experience, such as hot flashes, make that concept impractical.

Chemotherapy

Chemotherapy is not yet a major factor in prostate cancer treatment. Chemotherapy involves administration of highly potent drugs that lower the rate of cell growth within the body. When chemotherapy drugs are injected into the bloodstream, they circulate throughout the body and harm cancerous and healthy cells alike. However, the damage is greatest in the cells growing the fastest, including cancerous cells and those cells that govern hair growth.

To date, many chemotherapy drugs have been tested on prostate cancer. While many of them have been shown to be effective in treating other forms of cancer, so far none has proven very effective on prostate cancer. One problem may be the failure of many of them to effectively reach the prostate through the bloodstream. Chemotherapy drugs are also associated with many unpleasant side effects, including nausea, fatigue, body pain, and hair loss. Nonetheless, the possibility does exist that more effective prostate cancer chemotherapy agents will eventually be developed.

Hyperthermia

As discussed in Chapter 5, hyperthermia employing localized heat produced by microwaves has shown promise in treating benign prostate enlargement. Encouraging results are also indicated in some patients with certain types of prostate cancer. The advantage of effective hyperthermia in treating prostate cancer would be similar to that suggested for BPH, an easy-to-tolerate, nonsurgical procedure that can be performed as an outpatient.

Hyperthermia can kill cancer cells, increase a patient's ability to kill cancer cells, and increase the effect that either radiation therapy or chemotherapy drugs have on cancerous cells. Hyperthermia can also relieve many uncomfortable symptoms such as urinary obstruction or pain in the pelvis. In a few cases, men with cancer which has spread outside the prostate have enjoyed shrinking of the metastasized cancers, because of the boost that their immune systems received.

Immunotherapy

Immunotherapy strengthens the body's natural immune system. The human body has a built-in defense mechanism, operating through agents in the bloodstream that identifies and kills invading organisms. Being out of the ordinary, cancerous cells may appear to be undesirable invaders to the immune system.

In immunotherapy, certain drugs have been found to improve this identification and killing process. Considerable attention has centered on supplementation of a drug known as interleukin-2, a complex substance produced naturally by the body's immune system. This drug promotes the growth of additional immune cells in the bloodstream. Lymphokine-activated killer T cells are also being investigated.

Vaccines are also at an early stage of study and may prevent the recurrence of prostate and other cancers in patients who have previously been treated for malignancies. Tumor tissue is obtained by biopsy from an individual patient and a vaccine is produced in the laboratory that can later be injected into the patient. Thus, a potential exists for protecting a patient with a vaccine prepared from his own body.

So far, results with immunotherapy are limited and hopes should not be raised prematurely for a major new approach to treating cancer, including prostate cancer. Nevertheless, given the key role played by the immune system in disease prevention and control, this area of research has profound long-range promise.

Gene Therapy

Gene therapy in cancer treatment involves altering DNA, the basic chemical substance governing growth and function of every cell in your body. By using genetic engineering, the possibility exists to manufacture and introduce into the body new genes that may make cells more resistant to the triggering of cancer or that make cells better cancer fighters when a cancer gets underway.

While gene therapy is still in its early stage, in the long-run, the possibility may exist for an effective end to the prostate cancer problem. A development with major implications on gene therapy is the ongoing Genome Project. In this massive undertaking, scientists are mapping the entire DNA structure of the human body. Once completed, results may offer a workable means of pinpointing and altering areas associated with each type of cancer.

Watchful Waiting

Another controversial and very conservative strategy often amounts to no treatment at all. Called "watchful waiting," this strategy involves regularly monitoring the progress of the tumor and treating it only when necessary, such as to relieve specific symptoms like bone pain, or when urinary tract obstruction must be cleared by a TURP or other treatment.

Proponents of watchful waiting cite some studies which show long-term survival rates about the same in men who have been treated for prostate cancer versus men who have not been treated. Since prostate cancer is generally a very slow-progressing cancer which occurs most frequently in older men, the theory is that many older men can coexist with a certain amount of prostate cancer and will probably die of something else. Watchful waiting allows men to live without the side effects of other treatments, often with a higher quality of life, and with much less expense than other treatments.

A major disadvantage to watchful waiting is that it adds a lot of uncertainty to the treatment process, since treatment is reactive rather than aggressive. Watchful waiting may have value in some cases, such as in men over seventy with a predominantly nonaggressive tumor. But opponents of watchful waiting say this therapy has the dangerous potential of allowing a cancer which can be cured to grow to a stage where a cure is no longer possible. A localized malignant tumor in the prostate doubles in size about every two years. Watchful waiting could be very dangerous for relatively young men in high risk groups whose prostate cancer is discovered in the early stages, before prostate cancer has metastasized.

Patients must be presented with all the options for treatment by their urologist, including watchful waiting. Your age, your family responsibilities, and your financial situation are all variables to be considered. Since this is a stressful time for many patients, you may well ask your urologist to bring another professional such as a social worker or a psychologist into the decision-making process.

Appropriate Treatments at Each Stage of Prostate Cancer

This discussion identifies treatment programs employed most often at various stages of prostate cancer. You should be aware that because urologists often disagree about treatment, a variety of options exists for treatment at each stage of the disease.

In my practice, I take into consideration factors such as age, general health, possible effects on lifestyle, and the feelings of my fully informed patient before recommending any treatment program. A highly aggressive treatment designed for a fifty-five-year-old man in good physical condition will not necessarily be appropriate for a man of thirty in more fragile health.

Treating Stage A Prostate Cancer

Unfortunately, most prostate cancer is not discovered in Stage A. Therefore, urologists have limited experience in treating the disease at that stage, although that should improve with more effective early diagnosis.

When prostate cancer is discovered in Stage A, your urologist will likely recommend prompt radical prostatectomy for both Stages A_1 and A_2 treatment, especially if you are in reasonably good health and not much older than sixty. If you are older, your urologist may still recommend radical prostatectomy if you appear to be an acceptable operative risk generally based on good health, a positive attitude, and a strong desire to achieve a complete cure.

This preference for radical prostatectomy is based on the belief that it offers the best chance for a complete and lasting cure. Men whose cancers are discovered and treated in Stage A can normally look forward to enjoying many years of productive and active life. Moreover, the side effects after radical prostatectomy, including impotence and incontinence, are treatable.

In older men with limited life expectancy, the urologist and patient may decide merely to monitor the disease, understanding that death will occur from other causes well before the cancer can progress to the point where it becomes a burden to the patient. With men who are poor operative risks, or who, for psychological and other reasons, object to surgery, radiation and hormonal therapies may be considered.

Treating Stage B Prostate Cancer

Most urologists prefer radical prostatectomy for Stage B prostate cancer at both the B_1 and B_2 substages. As with Stage A, radical prostatectomy may not be employed in elderly men, those who are poor operative risks, and men who simply wish to avoid surgery. Radiation therapy will often be recommended for these men, with the possible exception, as in Stage A, of very elderly men who have limited life expectancy.

In all candor, I should mention that a still-to-be-resolved controversy exists among urologists between those advocating radical prostatectomy and those who prefer radiation therapy in Stage B treatment. Not surprisingly, surgeons tend to favor the former approach, radiotherapists the latter. Both sides point to impressive-sounding studies to support their positions. The old apples to oranges factor often comes up when comparing results of these studies. Most are based on information collected at a single research center whose scientists differ about many significant factors, including the types of patients treated, statistical designs and analyses, and supplementary treatment with drugs.

In some men, detailed studies of the location and physical character of the tumor may provide a sound medical reason for choosing either radical prostatectomy or radiotherapy. If that is not the case, I prefer to follow at this time the prevailing belief of most authorities: Radical prostatectomy offers the most effective and lasting cure for prostate cancer. Keep in mind, though, that advances in surgical techniques such as lasers are reducing the stress and the risk of radical prostatectomy. Advances in radioactive seeding as discussed earlier could alter my opinion in the future. If you have any doubts about your situation, you should obtain a second or even a third opinion about the need for surgery.

Hormonal therapy can be used in treating Stage B prostate cancer, sometimes combined with radical prostatectomy or radiation therapy. Some controversy exists in connection with such treatment. The case for hormonal drugs is strongest in Stage B men who, because of age and general health, are not good candidates for either radical prostatectomy or radiation therapy. The consensus of experts is that there is insufficient evidence that hormonal therapy provides significant benefits at Stage B. Moreover, hormonal therapy is costly and, as indicated, can have undesirable side effects. These disadvantages could change with new information and with the appearance of better drugs.

Treating Stage C Prostate Cancer

Most prostate cancer is first diagnosed at Stage C, in up to 40 percent of cases. Some cases may be diagnosed at an earlier stage, then progress to Stage C. Typically, treatment programs for Stage C prostate cancer attempt to control the growth of a malignant tumor in the prostate region, prevent spread of malignant cells to other parts of the body, and maximize the period in which the patient is free from unpleasant aspects of the disease.

Radical prostatectomy is often employed in Stage C to reduce the total number of malignant cells in the body, thus reducing the cancerous cells that can spread to other parts of the body as well as the burden on the body's immune system. However, not even radical prostatectomy in Stage C can be counted on to remove *all* cancerous cells from the body. Radiation therapy can also be used at Stage C in men who are not good candidates for radical prostatectomy.

Hormonal therapy is important in Stage C, often in combination with a radical prostatectomy. While similar to Stage B, there is incomplete agreement as to when to initiate hormonal treatment nor how aggressive it should be. Some urologists advocate hormonal treatment immediately after Stage C diagnosis, reasoning that the risks of delay outweigh the hormonal treatment burden on the patient. Other doctors reason that treatment is better delayed at least until radical prostatectomy or radiotherapy results can be evaluated. There is no simple answer to this question because the best treatment approach depends on how far the disease has spread and on the patient's individual needs and physical condition.

Hormonal therapy in Stage C still includes orchiectomy (castration) and estrogen administration. Lately, some attention has shifted to treatment with advanced drugs such as leuprolide and flutamine. These drugs are often used in combination. When a combination is effective, the patient benefits both from retarding the spread of the disease and by avoiding castration and the undesirable side effects of estrogen.

Treating Stage D Prostate Cancer

In Stage D prostate cancer, treatment emphasis is on prolonging life by preventing further spread of the disease and by providing relief from the disease symptoms. Immediate orchiectomy, owing to its usual effectiveness, is often recommended for patients whose condition is first diagnosed in Stage D. Combination therapy, with drugs like leuprolide and flutamine, is often tried. Goserelin acetate (Zoladex) is finding increasing favor for Stage D treatment. Radical prostatectomy is still employed to remove the primary tumor from the prostate in suitable Stage D patients.

Pain in the bones is one of the most unpleasant symptoms in Stage D prostate cancer. Various drugs can relieve this and other symptoms. Radiotherapy also has some role in reducing bone pain. One treatment being studied now and yielding promising results is radioactive strontium.

If You Have Prostate Cancer

For every one hundred men who are told they have Stage A prostate cancer, on average and with proper treatment, seventy-seven are still alive (often doing very well) five years later. With Stage B prostate cancer, sixty-five survive. At Stage C and Stage D prostate cancer, forty-eight C and twenty-one D men survive after five years.

To put these odds in better perspective, consider that with esophageal cancer, on average, only twenty men are alive after five years. With pancreatic cancer, only three survive after five years and most are dead six months after being diagnosed. Bear in mind when evaluating your chances that the odds with prostate cancer reflect, to an important extent, that nobody lives forever. Because prostate cancer in most men usually occurs late in life, a significant number of men with the disease will realize their allotted life expectancy, dying from other causes within the five-year period following diagnosis.

Furthermore, your chances may be even better than indicated if your general health is good and you cooperate with your treatment program. Good cardiovascular fitness, proper diet, exercise, and ideal body weight improve greatly your ability to withstand the inherent stress of radical prostate surgery, radiotherapy, and other prostate cancer treatments. Some of my patients are alive and living useful lives ten and fifteen years after prostate cancer was diagnosed.

Another important tip: The disease will probably have serious emotional consequences for you, your partner (should you have one), and for your close family members. Don't hesitate to discuss these issues with your urologist. You may want to consider joining a support group, such as those discussed in Chapter 11.

Remember, prostate cancer is curable or controllable. With effective treatment, most men can look forward to many more quality years. Early diagnosis is crucial.

Surgical prostate removal is still the preferred solution to prostate cancer treatment in its early and localized stages. Radiation therapy is a suitable alternative for some patients. With advanced prostate cancers, hormonal therapy is an effective treatment.

Prostate cancer treatment is continuing to improve as surgical and radiotherapy techniques advance and more effective drugs are developed. By the year 2000, hyperthermia, immunotherapy, and gene therapy may offer additional tools. At this time, government support for breast cancer research is about six times greater than for prostate cancer. This level of funding should improve, accelerating the pace of research given the evidence of growing public awareness and rising concerns.

Never think that a completely satisfactory sex life ends after you're treated for a prostate tumor. The next chapter deals with sexual issues.

CHAPTER 7

Prostate Treatment and Sex: Your Best Years Are Ahead

Impotence and a lack of sexual desire are two male sexual dysfunctions sometimes experienced as side effects of benign and malignant prostate tumor treatment. In benign prostate hyperplasias (BPH), impotence may be a consequence of both surgery and hormonal therapy. With prostate cancer, radiation therapy may be an additional contributing factor to impotence. Lack of sexual desire may be a consequence of hormonal therapy both in BPH and prostate cancer treatment.

Only about one-third of the urologists in the United States have made the treatment of impotence or male sexual problems an important part of their practice. One good way to locate a urologist who treats impotence is to call the urology department of a local hospital or medical school, and ask for a referral. In the yellow pages, urologists who specialize often advertise their treatment of sexual impotence. Other groups such as American Medical Systems Impotence Information Center hotline will provide a list of urologists in a particular geographic area who are currently diagnosing and treating impotence.

It is estimated that 60 percent of men who are impotent delay seeing a doctor for at least a year. Some men wait five or ten years before seeking help. There is no reason to delay, since the vast majority of men with impotence may be helped.

To help you understand better the impotency problem, this chapter describes how erection and ejaculation occur normally, then explains some factors that can adversely affect these natural processes. You'll find practical advice on the growing number of increasingly effective treatments for impotence followed by background on the causes of loss of sexual desire and how it can be treated.

Putting Impotence in Perspective

Impotence is the number one concern of most men who face prostate treatment, especially for those awaiting surgery. However, impotence is a complex medical problem and if you do experience it after prostate treatment, the treatment itself may not be the only cause or even the most important. Let's try to consider impotence within the overall perspective of prostate treatment.

Take David, a fifty-two-year-old lawyer. Several months after his BPH surgery, he came to my office for a routine follow-up examination. My standard practice is to ask postsurgical patients whether they have noticed any problems with sexual performance. After some hesitation, and obvious distress, David admitted he was having some difficulties. During the discussion that followed, David said he had been having frequent episodes of impotence for about two years before his prostate surgery.

Glancing over his medical records, I noticed he had not checked impotence as a problem on the questionnaire he filled out on his first visit, nor had he ever mentioned an ongoing problem in any of our talks before his operation. David's explanation was that he was too embarrassed to say anything. Erroneously, he associated his impotence with the enlarged prostate condition, hoping the surgery would somehow cure both problems.

After chiding him for not being entirely open with me about his medical background, I investigated his impotence further. David's problem had first appeared when he began to take a beta blocker medication for high blood pressure. His physician, an internist, had failed to mention impotence as a possible side effect of that drug. I suggested David talk to his internist, who switched David to an alternative drug of the calcium channel-blocker type. The new drug proved just as effective in treating his high blood pressure, but without imposing the impotence side effect.

This case is an important reminder that when a man tells his urologist he is experiencing difficulties with sexual performance after prostate treatment, it is not always the treatment underlying the problem. Of course, impotence is sometimes an unavoidable result of BPH treatment or prostate cancer regimes. BPH and prostate cancer treatment are often needed at a time in life when other factors can cause impotence. These alternative influences may be crucial in solving impotency. Always make it a point to tell your urologist before prostate treatment if you have any history of impotence. If you experience it for the first time following prostate treatment, ask your urologist to determine whether the problem may not be partially or entirely the result of an alternative cause, or have him refer you to a urologist who specializes in male sexual dysfunction.

Impotence and Its Causes

What Exactly Is Impotence?

Impotence is the inability of a man to obtain an erection of adequate rigidity to permit vaginal penetration and, once the penis is in position, to maintain erection long enough for the mutual satisfaction of both partners. Definitions are never perfect. As we pointed out in Chapter 4, some women need an extended period to achieve orgasm, or they may never achieve orgasm through conventional sexual intercourse. A man's inability to maintain an erection under those circumstances is *not* impotence. Chapter 4 also warned that attempts by a man to prolong intercourse unreasonably can cause an unpleasant prostate irritation. Therefore, if your partner has a problem achieving orgasm through conventional intercourse, you both have a responsibility to consider alternatives.

Impotence must also be distinguished from another form of male sexual dysfunction—premature ejaculation. In that situation, with minimal foreplay, the man obtains an adequate erection, but ejaculates before vaginal penetration or very shortly thereafter. By contrast, if you're impotent, foreplay will not result in an erection rigid enough for vaginal penetration, or one that remains firm enough for the man to achieve orgasm when inserted into the vagina.

Erectile dysfunction carries with it a great emotional wallop, since it is bound up with every man's feelings about himself. Some men try to go this problem alone, and don't involve their spouses in the medical advice they receive regarding erectile dysfunction. Other men may avoid sexual situations in an effort to forget about the problem. When they feel rejected, however, spouses or lovers may wonder if their mate is having an affair, or that he thinks they are no longer attractive. For a number of reasons, many doctors think that a couple's best chance for an approach that will benefit them both comes when the couple participates and works together.

A urologist who specializes in the treatment of impotence should be seen if you have difficulty in achieving erections in three out of four attempts. Also see the urologist if this condition has existed for longer than a month, if morning and spontaneous erections become less common, if it takes longer to achieve an erection than in the past, or if it's more difficult than before to have intercourse in certain sexual positions.

Impotence may be temporary or chronic. Occasional episodes of erectile failure are common to all men. For example, under the influence of alcohol, men often experience temporary performance difficulties. Uncomfortable or threatening surroundings may also inhibit performance. If you experience any of these, don't conclude that you have a chronic impotence problem unless your failure to obtain an adequate erection occurs frequently, consistently, and under otherwise ideal surroundings. Occasionally, impotence may be caused by a history of diabetes, or be a result of medications prescribed to treat other ailments such as high blood pressure or depression. If a patient is reacting to a particular drug, switching to another medication can result in improvement.

If you do have chronic impotence, you are not alone. About one out of eight American men eventually develops chronic impotence. It affects men from all walks of life and is experienced regardless of ethnic or racial background. Impotence is also a growing health problem, owing to the aging of America's population. But just because impotence is associated with aging doesn't mean you have to accept the idea that your sex life will end as you grow older.

What Causes Impotence?

Until recently, most people believed impotence in younger men was mainly psychological. Failure to obtain an erection was thought to result from feelings of shame, guilt, and fear of sex, often repressed since childhood. Although many persons, surprisingly including some physicians, still believe impotence is largely "all in your head," it has become increasingly evident that most of the time it can be traced to a physical cause, or a combination of physical causes. In fact, now it is believed as many as 75 percent of all cases stem from physical, not psychological, factors. Psychological factors can be important, though, and some serious psychological problems can be the *result*, if not the *cause* of impotence.

The purely physical factors fall into two broad categories: abnormalities in the vascular system that supplies blood to and from the penis, and abnormalities in the nervous system that control the erection process. Let's take a look at how the normal processes of erection and ejaculation function.

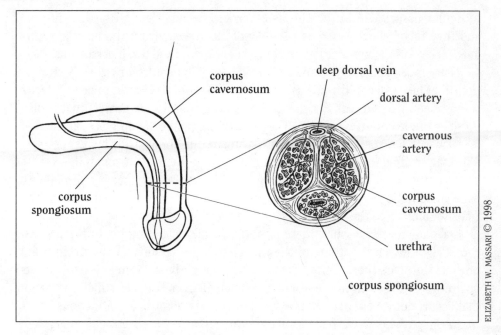

Figure 7.1 *Cross-section of the Penis*

In effect, the penis is a highly sophisticated hydraulic device. Two parallel cylin-drically-shaped erectile tissue structures, each known as "corpus cavernosum" (plural, "corpus cavernosa"), are located along two sides of the penis, extending from the base to a point near the tip. Inside each corpus cavernosum are thousands of tiny and expandable sac-shaped cavities known as sinuses, which can temporarily absorb and store quite large volumes of blood (see Figure 7.1). Any liquid is difficult to compress, so when these sinuses fill with blood, a buildup of pressure occurs along the outer shell of each sinus cavity. The result is the physical expansion and stiffening of these corpus cavernosa, or an erection.

For this hydraulic system to work, there must be a physical structure that traps blood within the corpus cavernosa. This is believed to be accomplished by a combination of increased blood flow to the corpus cavernosa and a valving action within them. The erection may begin when arteries supplying the erectile tissue of the penis dilate. This dilation (an increase in the diameter of the arteries) re-sults in increased flow of blood. As the erection process continues, the smooth muscular tissues within the corpus cavernosa become less tense than normal, and they relax, which restricts the flow of blood away from the erectile tissue. Feedback relationships are thought to exist between these two mechanisms.

There must also be some means for directing and controlling the physical actions that take place in the penis during erection. For an erection to occur, electrical messages have to pass through the nervous system to the centers that control muscles in the corpus cavernosa. These messages can be of two types. In the first, foreplay with a sexual partner or even viewing or imagining erotic images can send a message calling for an erection from the brain to the penis through the somatic nervous system. In the second, stroking the penis can send a message through the parasympathetic nervous system from nerve centers in the spinal column that transmit directly to the penis.

Ejaculation occurs when there is sufficient physical stimulus to the penis to cause vigorous contractions of the muscles in the vicinity of the urethra and prostate. In effect, these contractions squeeze out of the body, in a series of spurts, quantities of semen from the ejaculatory duct. Orgasm, the pleasurable sensation that occurs during ejaculation, is associated with these muscle contractions.

In Chapter 4, you learned ejaculation can occur in the absence of an erection. In other words, a man can be impotent in the sense of being unable to achieve or sustain vaginal penetration, but still ejaculate by masturbation, albeit with difficulty. Keep that in mind when reviewing treatments for impotence later in this chapter, in particular penile implants. They merely provide the stiffness necessary for vaginal penetration; by no means do they detract from the "natural" aspects or the physical pleasures of sexual intercourse.

Impotence Caused by a Vascular Problem

Impotence can be experienced when an abnormality causes insufficient blood flow into the penis. It also can occur when the internal valving mechanism is somehow defective and prevents blood flow out of the penis during the erectile process.

Insufficient blood flow into the penis can be caused by a buildup of fatty deposits known as plaque in the arteries supplying blood to the penis. The tiny size of these arteries, some with diameters smaller than a pin head, makes them vulnerable to plaque blockage. Plaque in the penile arteries is only one manifestation of arteriosclerosis, commonly known as hardening of the arteries. In that connection, men with a history of coronary heart disease—where plaque also plays a role—often report impotence.

Plaque formation is known to be associated with diets high in fats, especially too much cholesterol. Tobacco, particularly cigarettes, can exacerbate an impotence problem caused by plaque buildup in the penile arteries. Some substances in tobacco are known to constrict the penile arteries, further impeding blood flow. In fact, men sometimes report improved sexual performance after they stop smoking.

Besides plaque, there are other causes for blood restriction into the penis. Physical injury in the pelvic area, malignant tumors, or surgery performed on major blood vessels elsewhere in the body can cause blood clots to form, which dislodge the small fatty deposits present in the bloodstream. When these fragments, or emboli, flow downstream, penile arteries are one of the places they may end up.

When the valving mechanism designed to hold blood inside the penis during sexual activity fails to work properly, a continuous leakage of blood will occur through the veins that normally carry blood out of the penis, resulting in erections of insufficient rigidity or a quick loss of an erection. Later in this chapter, you'll discover medical science may be close to explaining the chief cause for this type of impotence.

One interesting condition is known as the "steal syndrome." Some men easily obtain erections during foreplay, but they disappear after intercourse is initiated. This problem is believed to result from a loss of blood from the penis as the level of physical activity increases during intercourse. In effect, blood is "stolen" from the penis in order to supply increased energy needs. Sometimes the steal syndrome can be overcome when intercourse is performed in a position requiring less exertion by the man, such as with the women on top. Other men find it easier to have intercourse standing up. To help sustain an erection, a soft tourniquet using a material called Coban may be wrapped around the base of the penis before attempting sexual activity—the tourniquet doesn't stop blood from flowing into the penis, only out.

Impotence Caused by a Nervous System Problem

Any serious breakdown at any point in the nerve circuits will make erection impossible. Physical injury to critical nerves in the spinal column, for example, is a frequent cause of impotence. Critical nerves can also be impaired by excessive use of alcohol; by taking certain illegal substances, especially cocaine and crack; by diabetes; kidney disease; and various neurological disorders, including multiple sclerosis and Parkinson's disease. The nervous system is also the pathway by which psychological factors may affect sexual performance.

Certain prescription and over-the-counter drugs can also result in impotence. Drugs prescribed for treatment of high blood pressure (hypertension), heart disease, and other cardiovascular problems are among those implicated most frequently. Some widely prescribed drugs of this type linked to impotence are Aldomet (methylodopa), Diuril (chlorothiazide), Inderal (propranolol), Lopressor (metoprolol), and Serpasil (reserpine). Generally, cardiovascular drugs of the beta-blocker type tend to be implicated most often. In contrast, the calcium channel-blocker drugs are associated with lesser side effects and are usually just as effective.

Impotence has also been linked to tranquilizers, antidepressants, and other drugs that control the emotions. Some well-known drugs in these categories that have been linked to impotence include Equanil (meprobamate), Elavil (amitriptyline), Haldol (haloperidol), Librium (chlordiazepoxide), and Valium (diazepam). Tagamet (cimetidine) and other drugs frequently prescribed for ulcers and other gastrointestinal problems are also associated with impotence. Some of the many other drugs linked to impotence include Dilantin (phenytoin) for treating seizures, Diamox (acetozolamide), used to treat glaucoma, and Larodopa (levodopa), to treat Parkinson's disease. As discussed in previous chapters, impotence can also be a consequence of the drugs used for hormonal treatment of prostatic tumors.

Many drugs available without prescription have been linked to impotence, too. These include many widely advertised drugs for treating the common cold and various allergies, and sleeping pills.

Fortunately, impotence often disappears when use of many of these drugs is discontinued and an alternative is substituted. Never discontinue a needed prescribed drug, however, without consulting your physician. It is always a good idea to inquire about the possibility of impotence whenever your physician prescribes any drug. In general, physicians are becoming more informed about impotence, but many still fail to take it into account when prescribing medication.

Impotence Caused by a Combination of Factors

When impotence is experienced after prostate treatment, more than one factor may be the cause. In prostate surgery, there may be significant damage to a key bundle of erection-control nerves in the prostate area. Surgery may also cause damage to important blood vessels supplying the penis. These problems can also result from bladder and rectal surgery. Radiation therapy for treating bladder and prostate cancer can cause considerable tissue scarring in the vicinity of the prostate that may impair nerve connections as well as blood flow.

Impotence can result from more than one factor in diabetes and kidney disease. About 50 percent of men with diabetes eventually experience impotence, usually after lesions form in the penile arteries. Later, the disease causes damage to the nerve pathways that control the penis. Kidney disease can cause nerve damage and abnormal hormonal levels that adversely affect erection.

Treating Impotence

Effective treatments are available in situations with a physical cause. The following section includes treatment based on drugs, penile implants, reconstructive surgery, and the use of vacuum devices. Some consideration is also given to the role of psychotherapy and sex therapy in impotence treatment.

Drugs for Treating Impotence

The search for a magic cure for impotence is as old as history and has so far yielded very few good results. Over the years, countless men have been taken in by "snake oil" salesmen who peddle worthless and sometimes dangerous products. The African rhinoceros has been driven almost to extinction, owing to the weird belief in the Far East that ingesting powdered rhinoceros horn creates extraordinary sexual vigor. Recently, as the medical profession has finally taken an interest in impotence, drugs that actually do help have been developed. All these drugs work by causing the blood vessels in the penis to dilate, which causes the penis to engorge with blood. The recent FDA approval of Viagra (sildenafil) marks a new era in the treatment of impotence. After a thorough medical history and physical examination, Viagra can be a firstline treatment. Viagra works by enhancing smooth muscle relaxation, allowing blood to enter and pool in the penis and creating an erection. Viagra can be taken thirty minutes to four hours before sexual activity. Major contraindications include men taking nitrates for the treatment of heart disease. Side effects reported include headaches, flushing, upset stomach, nasal congestion, and vision complaints.

Testosterone sometimes improves sexual performance. Its use, for reasons stated earlier, is precluded for men with benign prostate enlargement or prostate cancer. When taken under proper medical supervision, the hormone is of potential value in treating men with abnormally low levels of testosterone who have no evidence of prostate tumors. When testosterone treatment is indicated, the best way to take it is with intermuscular injections, or by implantation under the skin of small, slow-release testosterone pellets.

Yohimbine is an interesting drug first obtained from the dried bark of an African tree. Yohimbine helps impotence in some cases, particularly for diabetics. It has not been very effective on men who have had prostate treatment. The most common commercial product containing yohimbine on the market also contains methyltestosterone, so this product is not suitable for men with prostate tumors.

The most effective drugs for treating impotence are injected directly into the penis. They may help some men who became impotent from prostate treatment. Drugs injected directly into the penis have one advantage: Their pharmaceutical activity is limited mainly to the penis, not the entire body. Their disadvantages are discomfort and the possible psychological trauma of penile injection.

Penile injection therapy made its appearance during the eighties. Today, this approach is approved by the American Urological Association. The first drug to be widely used for penile injection was papaverine, which acts as a muscle relaxant and vasodilator. Papaverine has since been largely replaced by another drug, prostaglandin E_1, sold under the name Caverject. In 1995, the FDA approved Caverject for treatment of erectile dysfunction. A doctor's prescription is needed to obtain the product. Caverject is presently sold in sterile powder form, which is injected into the body with a short, thin hypodermic needle. With the injection, most men feel only a little pinch.

The drug takes effect in five to twenty minutes. Other, easier-to-use spring-loaded injection devices may soon appear on the market. According to published reports, the product works on 80 percent of men with erectile dysfunction. One long-term side effect is fibrosis or scarring of the skin, which occurs in 3 to 7 percent of men in studies. The most common short-term side effect (37 percent in clinical studies) is short-term penile pain.

When prostaglandin E_1 is injected directly into the penis using a hypodermic syringe, the usual result is an impressive erection that is highly suitable for sexual activities. Men who employ penile injection therapy using prostaglandin E_1 or any alternative drug must undergo a period of experimentation under the direction of a urologist specializing in the field. These studies are essential in order to determine proper dosage. Improper dosage can result in a condition resembling priapism, a dangerous condition characterized by persistent and painful erection.

During the study procedure, dosage is adjusted until a level is achieved that results in an erection lasting about forty-five minutes. During the study procedure, men are also taught how to inject themselves properly. Most men, including those who have experienced treatment for prostate conditions, are able to learn how to inject themselves at home with a minimum of discomfort and subsequently to engage in satisfactory sexual intercourse. The sensation of the injection has been described as a slight "pinch."

Penile injection therapy requires continuing medical supervision. The urologist will usually provide a supply of prefilled hypodermic syringes. Because of the possibility of irritation and scarring, penile injection should be used no more than twice a week with a gap of several days between each use.

Besides prostaglandin E_1 and papaverine, several other drugs are available for penile injection. Phentoamine is sold under the name Regitine. A newer drug, VIP, shows considerable promise, but is not generally available. These drugs are sometimes substituted for prostaglandin E_1 in men where that drug has undesirable side effects or when it has lost its effectiveness after extended use.

Penile Implants

Penile implants are prostheses implanted surgically within the penis, resulting in an erection of sufficient rigidity to engage in normal sexual intercourse. A prosthesis is any mechanical device that replaces a nonworking or missing part of the body. Using a penile implant to overcome impotence is no different than using a dental plate or wearing glasses.

Penile implants have been used for more than twenty years and have been found safe and effective. A man with an implant can fully experience satisfactory sex, including ejaculation and orgasm. He can also father children. Women find the sexual experience with a man with an implant satisfactory and completely natural.

Penile implants for men who become impotent after prostate treatment are highly appropriate. In fact, men whose impotence results from prostate surgery are among the second largest group that has chosen implants to solve their problem.

Implants are available in three basic designs, each of which has pluses and minuses. The semirigid malleable implant is the simplest, with the advantage of being the least expensive, in terms of the device itself as well as associated surgical and hospitalization cost. This implant is essentially a rod-shaped device made from silicone. With the implant inside the penis, it can be straightened out into the normal erectile position before intercourse. Then, the implant provides adequate rigidity for successful intercourse. However, there is no increase in penis length or girth. After intercourse, the penis can be bent down close to the body. The disadvantage of the semirigid malleable implant is that there is some degree of permanent erection. Although it is unnoticeable under loose-fitting clothing, it can be a problem to some men in locker-room situations.

The most expensive device in terms of overall cost is the three-piece inflatable implant. This device, mainstay of most implanted men, incorporates two parallel hollow cylinders placed inside the penis, a pump and valve mechanism inserted into the scrotum, and a spherical reservoir containing hydraulic fluid inserted into the lower abdomen. To obtain an erection, the owner simply squeezes the pumping mechanism he can easily feel inside his scrotum, which causes fluid to flow from the reservoir into the two cylinders, thus producing an erection. After intercourse, the device is easily deflated and the penis returns to its normal, flaccid state.

The chief advantage of the three-piece implant is that it provides the most authentic-looking erection possible and one that includes increased penis length and girth. Besides its higher cost, installation of the three-piece inflatable implant requires a more complicated surgical procedure. More can go wrong once it's in place, thus necessitating a follow-up surgical procedure. However, I have done several thousand three-piece implants in my practice, and can advise that any urologist who performs the surgery frequently should be able to install the device in less than forty-five minutes. In a recent analysis of the postsurgical experience over a fourteen-year period, patients further reveal only a 1 percent infection rate and a 3 percent rate of mechanical failure.

The third device is a simple, self-contained inflatable implant, which represents a compromise between the semirigid malleable implant and the three-piece inflatable implant in overall cost and performance. This device consists of two parallel cylinders, each of which contains hydraulic fluid. When the cylinders are in place, an erection can easily be obtained by squeezing the ends of the cylinder near the front of the penis. One advantage of the self-contained inflatable implant over the three-piece inflatable one is that no components need be implanted inside the scrotum or abdomen. Its erection is not as full, nor is there any increase in penile length and girth as with the three-piece inflatable implant. But compared to the semirigid malleable implant, it provides a controllable erection and the penis will usually return to a fully flaccid state when the device is deflated.

For men who experience both impotence and incontinence after prostate treatment, both a penile implant and an artificial urinary sphincter can be installed. This latter device, described in the following chapter, is often an effective solution to incontinence. Depending on its type, your section of the country, and whether surgery is performed in a hospital or as an outpatient, overall cost for a penile implant could range from under $10,000 to about $20,000. Concerns about silicone breast implants do not apply with penile implants. The principal problem in the former was leakage of liquid silicone material. The hydraulic fluid in penile implants is mainly sterile water.

Within two or three weeks after surgery, most men don't have physical discomfort with any of these devices. Most say the device just becomes like another part of their body, and they don't realize it's there unless they think about it.

If impotence is a likely result of surgery, patients have found that a simultaneous placement of penile implants during radical prostatectomy results in faster sexual rehabilitation, according to an article in the *Journal of Urology.* The surgery took an additional hour and a half. In a survey of men in Boston who had the procedure done, twenty out of twenty-two were sexually active within three months, a much higher rate than normal.

In my practice, I conduct a continuing mail questionnaire survey of patients who have had implants. Over 90 percent of my past patients report satisfactory results. However, an implant does involve a major surgical procedure, which may not be appropriate for some patients. There is also the cost, although there is usually adequate coverage in most medical insurance policies. You should not decide to have an implant until fully discussing your options with a urologist who specializes in impotence, and with your partner.

Reconstructive Surgery

Reconstructive surgery is just beginning to be important in treating impotence. So far, the results are mixed, with reconstructive surgery appropriate mainly in younger men with straddle-type injuries.

These surgical procedures involve either correcting insufficient blood flow into the penis or blood leaking out of the penis. Obstacles to inward blood flow are located with ultrasound imaging. These obstacles can include lesions caused by cardiovascular disease or scar tissue from physical injury. They are removed surgically.

One alternative has been to create an arterial bypass around the obstructed area, but you should be cautious about this surgery. Considerable current concern exists regarding the effectiveness of all arterial bypass surgery, but especially in treating heart disease. In coronary arterial bypass surgery, the installed bypass usually closes on its own within ten years. In penile arterial bypasses, the closure can take place in as few as six months.

When correcting leakage, the source of the leak in the veins that drain blood from the penis is first located with a special X-ray test called a corpus cavernosagram. Once located, the leak is sutured. By contrast with arterial surgery, this procedure can be performed under local anesthesia, often as an outpatient. However, this procedure is not always effective and requires the professional services of a highly specialized urologist, rather than a general urologist.

Unfortunately, there is little that can yet be done surgically to repair nerves damaged during prostate surgery or by radiation therapy. However, surgery may help some men who are impotent after prostate treatment, provided there is evidence that a vascular problem is a contributing factor.

Vacuum and Other External Devices

External devices employing a partial vacuum to help a man obtain an erection have grown more important recently. Once sold mainly in sex and novelty shops, these devices have become more sophisticated and have thus gained medical acceptance. Purchasing the better vacuum devices now requires a physician's prescription.

In one device, before sexual intercourse the man places his penis inside a condom-shaped chamber. With a pump, a vacuum is created around the penis. This vacuum draws blood into the penis, thus establishing an erection. Pressure at the base of the penis maintains the erection for a sufficient period of time.

Vacuum devices are a relatively simple and noninvasive approach to treating impotence. Reportedly, they have helped some men and are generally considered safe. However, some men find them ineffective and unpleasant. One of my patients described the device he tried as a "barbaric torture chamber."

Penile constriction rings are another external device. They fit tightly around the base of the penis and provide some degree of rigidity for intercourse. The stability of the erection is not always acceptable, however, because the constriction ring hardens only the outer, visible two-thirds of the penis. The erection might wobble, but it's adequate for penetration. There can be some discomfort on the skin of the penis due to the vacuum, but most men get used to this. Although the success rate is between 70 and 80 percent, not many men choose this device. Always use penile constriction rings with considerable caution, because there is a real possibility of injury if the penis swells up and makes the ring impossible to remove.

Psychotherapy and Sex Therapy

In traditional psychotherapy, impotence along with other forms of sexual dysfunction is treated typically with what is known as "talk therapy," an extended series of forty-five- to fifty-minute sessions during which the patient is encouraged to relate freely with the therapist past and current events, personal feelings, the content of dreams, and so forth. Talk therapy is based on the premise that by recalling and understanding early emotional experiences that underlie sexual dysfunctions, the patient will be relieved of the problem. This treatment is expensive, requires a strong commitment, and can extend over many years.

Contemporary sex therapy is less ambitious and concentrates on the specific dysfunction. Many sex therapists employ the "sensate focus" approach or some variation of it as developed by Masters and Johnson during the sixties. Typically, this approach consists of a short, highly intensive program of specially designed sexual exercises, educational seminars, and interactive discussions. Male and female partners are encouraged to participate together, but when a partner is unavailable, a surrogate may be provided.

The limited number of scientific studies of the effectiveness of psychotherapy and sex therapy in treating impotence show mixed success. Treatment is most successful when the impotence is purely psychological. Obviously, that is not the case with men who are impotent from the side effects of prostate treatment.

However, impotence can be very emotionally damaging and can cause serious problems in the relationship between men and their partners. In some cases, psychotherapy and sex therapy are useful in treating the emotional consequences of impotence and possibly alleviating the symptoms when the physical causes are minor. Before embarking on any program of psychotherapy or sex therapy on your own, consult your urologist.

Treating Lack of Desire

Lack of desire is the complete or nearly complete absence of sexual interest, and it may exist even in men who are fully capable of sexual performance. It is a biological fact that sexual interest, otherwise known as libido, is the normal state of all healthy adult males. Unless there are factors at work that repress the libido, virtually all adult men, regardless of moral upbringing and age, experience frequent erotic mental images. Reproduction is essential to the survival of the species and these images are part of the human survival strategy programmed into your DNA. For its own protection, however, society places restrictions on overt male sexual behavior.

If you experience lack of desire, you should regard the condition as abnormal, deserving of professional investigation. Be sure you tell your urologist about the problem. Lack of desire is a condition that lowers your quality of life and it has the potential to damage personal relationships. It also may be a symptom of a physical problem requiring treatment.

Often, lack of desire is caused by low levels of testosterone. Therefore, men who need hormonal therapy for treatment of benign or malignant prostate tumors or who have had to undergo an orchiectomy often experience it. However, lack of desire is complicated and clearly, psychological factors are often at work.

Normally, testosterone levels are not affected by transurethral resection or by radical prostatectomy. However, lack of desire can occur in men after these operations, even absent simultaneous treatment with hormonal therapy. Under those circumstances, the problem may be psychological and possibly treatable with routine counseling. In Chapter 8, you'll learn incontinence is a problem with highly emotional consequences that sometimes follows prostate treatment. The fear an incontinent man has of being embarrassed while engaging in sexual activities is one factor that can impact sexual desire. Another is a condition called "performance anxiety," when a man is afraid to attempt sexual activites. In some men, this condition may be connected with the mistaken belief that prostate surgery automatically ends a man's sexual capability.

Several physical disorders that should not be ruled out when lack of desire follows prostate surgery include postoperative infections of the urethra and the prostate that sometimes occur after prostate surgery and may result in premature and painful ejaculation. Under those circumstances, lack of desire is quite understandable. Hyperthyroidism and kidney disorders are two other possible physical conditions that sometimes cause lack of desire. Treating these conditions may help solve a libido problem.

Your Best Sexual Years Are Ahead

If you are facing treatment for BPH or prostate cancer, there is no reason not to believe your best sexual years are still ahead. Although new nerve-sparing surgical techniques are not always completely effective, they offer the promise of a decreased incidence of impotence that will probably improve further. Research now underway in neurosurgery may permit in the not too distant future the effective restoration of nerves damaged unavoidably during prostate surgery.

Despite impressive recent medical advances, impotence is sometimes unavoidably experienced after prostate treatment. This chapter has examined all the known causes of impotence, pointing out the need to examine the broad picture when dealing with any impotence problem after prostate treatment. This is essential because BPH and prostate cancer treatment occurs most often at a time in life when multiple factors can be operating.

Impotence is known to be caused mainly by physical factors—defects in the vascular system, in the nerve circuits controlling erection, or a combination of both. When impotence follows prostate treatment, a combination of factors is usually involved.

Effective means are available to help men who are impotent as a result of prostate treatment. At this time, penile injections and penile implants are the most appropriate. You should discuss them with your urologist and, if necessary, request a referral to a urologist who specializes in male sexual dysfunction.

The next chapter describes two other possible side effects of prostate treatment—incontinence and infertility. As with impotence, effective solutions are available.

CHAPTER 8

Coping with Incontinence and Infertility

Both incontinence and infertility are possible complications after treatment for benign prostatic hyperplasia (BPH) and prostate cancer either with surgery or radiation therapy. Both conditions can be treated effectively.

Incontinence and infertility are covered together in this chapter because after impotence they represent the second and third most frequently expressed concerns of my patients and because these two problems can be related. Infertility attributable to prostate infection is also discussed in this chapter.

Incontinence and the Prostate

Types of Prostate-Related Incontinence

Broadly defined, incontinence is the loss of voluntary control over passing waste products from the bladder and less commonly from the bowel. Here, we'll deal only with urinary incontinence, the inability to consciously control urine flow from the bladder.

Incontinence associated with prostate treatment may be either temporary or permanent. Temporary incontinence and occasional passage of blood in the urine happen to almost all patients after they have prostate surgery. As they heal, incontinence and bleeding often go away, sometimes while they're still in the hospital or within a few weeks after they get home.

Unless your urologist observes strong indications to the contrary, never conclude you are permanently incontinent unless your condition persists and shows no signs of diminishing for at least six months after transurethral resection, radical prostatectomy, or radiation treatment. With modern techniques, your chances of permanent incontinence are no more than 1.5 percent in the case of a TURP, and 2 percent with radical prostatectomy. Following radiation therapy, your chances of incontinence are typically less than 5 percent.

Total incontinence is common after a prostatectomy, but it usually goes away within a year. A majority of men experience incontinence for the first 3 to 6 months after a radical prostatectomy. About 75 percent are continent after six months, and 90 to 95 percent are continent after one year.

Incontinence can have several different forms. But following prostate surgery, it is usually of the "urgency" type, occurring when there is a sudden, uninhibited contraction of the bladder. Urgency incontinence gives you virtually no warning of the impending expulsion of urine, so you have no time to reach the bathroom.

More than half of all incontinence cases in both men and women are believed to be "stress" incontinence, a condition somewhat less serious than urgency, and characterized by the insignificant loss of urine following laughter, coughing, lifting heavy objects, or straining the body physically in other ways. Men may experience some degree of stress incontinence after prostate treatment, but not as severe as urgency incontinence.

Some men may experience a condition known as "overflow" incontinence, sometimes known as "paradoxical" incontinence, characterized by the frequent, temporary inability to void when the need is apparent, followed by uncontrollable urine flow. Typically, the flow is at a slower rate than is the case with urgency incontinence. Overflow incontinence is a condition that can be caused by prostate enlargement and is not a consequence of surgical or radiation prostate treatment. If you experience symptoms of overflow incontinence, you should consult a urologist.

Two other conditions are "functional" and "iatrogenic" incontinence. The former occurs when men are unable to make it to the bathroom on time owing to physical injury or psychological problems, a condition common among older men confined in nursing homes. The iatrogenic form is associated with drugs, including certain antihistamines, heart disease and blood pressure medications, tranquilizers, and muscle relaxants. Men who have had surgical or radiation prostate treatment may experience either functional or iatrogenic incontinence, but not usually because of prostate treatment.

Problems of Incontinent Men

Problems associated with incontinence include inconvenience, discomfort, and hygienic consequences, all manageable and sometimes curable, so normally there should be no physical reason keeping you from living a full and active life if you should become incontinent after prostate treatment. Unfortunately, many men have a hard time coping with the emotional consequences of incontinence.

Homer, a fifty-year-old commercial photographer, became permanently incontinent after transurethral resection. He had been a good patient, but when the permanence of his condition became apparent, he became increasingly depressed, did his best to avoid all social contact, and began to drink heavily.

Discussing his problem with Homer, I learned he had been raised in a very authoritarian home where bedwetting was a point of great contention. His parents had tried to toilet train Homer well before the age of two and he still remembered being shamed by his parents after frequent accidents.

In treating him, I had to address both Homer's emotional and his physical difficulties. He benefited almost at once when I told him his childhood bedwetting was not his fault, nor was it a disgrace. Surgical implantation of an artificial urinary sphincter resulted in effective physical control of Homer's incontinence. In a few months, Homer's emotional state had improved greatly and he was enjoying a fully acceptable lifestyle.

Homer is not unusual. Despite a trend toward more enlightened attitudes, society still places a premium on early toilet training and regards a child's incontinence as a failing. Consider the popular conservative radio talk show host who uses the term "bedwetter" as a pejorative, someone akin to a wimp, or maybe a liberal.

If you do experience prostate-related incontinence, it will definitely help you if you are familiar with the connection between any early and aggressive toilet training and your emotional reaction as an incontinent adult. Everybody is incontinent at birth, but by age three, most children are well on their way to bladder control, with only minimal effort by their parents. In fact, most physicians will not conclude a childhood incontinence problem actually exists until loss of bladder control occurs daily well past three. However, occasional mishaps are normal to all young children. Pushing toilet training too early and making too much fuss over an occasional mishap may instill a feeling of guilt and shame in a young child that can last a lifetime.

It may also help to put in proper perspective the issues of spreading disease and giving offense. Contrary to popular belief, urine is normally sterile and, absent of any infectious microorganisms, will *not* spread disease. Also, urine will not smell unless there is infection or some other abnormality. But urine can be dark yellow, which may make accidental staining of your underwear and trousers more apparent. Dark-colored urine usually results from drinking insufficient water. Dark urine sometimes scares incontinent men into drastically limiting their water intake in the mistaken belief that it will help alleviate their condition.

The Extent of Incontinence

Incontinence affects an estimated 20 million men and women in the United States and Canada. Although the success rate in treating all types of urinary incontinence is about 80 percent, it is estimated that only one in twelve incontinent people ever seeks help which adds considerable uncertainty to the estimates. Of course, many individuals have only borderline symptoms and do not bother to seek help, and when they do, there is a question whether their symptoms should be classed as permanent incontinence.

Among American men, prostate treatment is an important element in permanent incontinence. There are no hard figures, but some estimates suggest as many as 1.5 to 2 million American men may have a permanent incontinence problem, possibly related to prostate surgery or radiation therapy. On that basis, prostate surgery could be a factor in about a fourth of all incontinence cases in adult males. As discussed below, there may also be multiple causes.

Treating adult incontinence in the United States has become a growth industry. If you doubt that, just watch primetime televison some evening and see if there aren't several commercials for adult incontinence products. The number of incontinent individuals is growing, owing to the continuing upward trend in the average age of Americans. The relative importance of prostate treatment in the overall incontinence picture will probably decline though, as improved surgical and radiation techniques continue to be developed.

How Prostate Treatment Can Cause Incontinence

To see how prostate surgery may result in incontinence, let's take a quick look at human urinary plumbing. In both men and women, the urinary process begins in the kidneys, a pair of vital organs whose main function is to purify your blood. Blood flows continuously into each of your two kidneys through the large artery known as the aorta. Once inside the kidneys, blood is filtered and any impurities are removed. The purified blood is recirculated into the bloodstream. Roughly 10 percent of the fluid volume of blood entering the kidneys becomes urine that carries these filtered impurities outside your body. Urine exits from each kidney and flows to the bladder through two ducts called ureters.

In effect, the bladder is a storage tank that holds a continuously increasing volume of urine until a buildup of pressure sends a signal to your brain indicating the need to void. At the base of the bladder is the urethra, the pipeline that carries urine outside your body. In men, this outlet passes first through the prostate and then through the penis. In both men and women, two circular muscles known as sphincters serve as valves that control urine flow from the bladder. If all is well, the valves close normally and urine is retained until voiding is socially convenient. When you are ready to void, your brain sends a message through the somatic or conscious nerve circuits ordering the valves to open and then you can urinate.

The average adult male passes about one quart of urine a day. Over an average lifetime, that adds up to somewhat more liquid than would fill a standard, aboveground, eighteen-foot-diameter swimming pool. Given the amount of work performed constantly by your urinary system, it is hardly surprising that some form of trouble, like incontinence, may eventually occur.

In men, incontinence can be caused by a number of factors: prostate enlargement, diabetes, spinal-cord injuries, spina bifida, strokes, multiple sclerosis, certain drugs, and other conditions that impair the critical sections of the nervous system controlling voiding. Proper function of the urinary sphincter muscles is sometimes impaired by physical injury, urinary infections, or by an obstruction at the bladder outlet. Muscle function may also decline over the years from the natural aging process. In some incontinent individuals, psychological factors may also be present.

When incontinence follows prostate treatment, the usual cause is surgical damage to the urinary sphincter muscles, impairment of the nerves controlling sphincter action, or some combination of both. The anatomy around the prostate is very crowded so that, even with the most advanced surgical techniques, avoiding some damage to nearby healthy tissues during a transurethral or radical prostatectomy is almost unavoidable.

When prostate treatment causes serious damage to the sphincter, it usually remains fully or partially open. A constant dripping form of incontinence is a typical result. As might be expected, the leak tends to be especially bad when standing or sitting, tapering somewhat when you lie down.

Most men who require major prostate surgery are usually of an age when there is a strong possibility of incontinence from causes other than surgery. In my practice, I always investigate the bigger picture because some factor other than surgical damage may contribute to the problem. The condition may be caused or complicated by a so-called irritable bladder, a neurological problem. Under those circumstances, treating that additional factor may result in a marked improvement in the patient's condition. Simple tests can diagnose many of the additional factors that may contribute to incontinence.

Managing Incontinence After Prostate Treatment

With the many methods now available to manage incontinence, effective solutions are possible for every patient.

Absorbent Products

Absorbent products are the most common way to deal with incontinence. They are easy to use, readily available, and fairly inexpensive.

A number of absorbent products on the market are designed to be worn under normal street clothing. For men with a minor incontinence problem, a drip collector (a pouchlike device worn over the penis) may be sufficient. Shields, a product resembling a feminine menstrual pad, are designed for individuals with light to moderate loss of bladder control. Adult undergarments are products like diapers and are intended for individuals with moderate to severe control loss. For those with either minimal or complete loss, a fitted garment known as a brief, resembling regular underpants, is also available.

All these products have their pluses and minuses, including varying degrees of comfort and protection, ease of disposability, and how convenient it may be to carry an adequate supply while engaging in normal activities. Recently, there has been fierce competition between two well-known companies, Kimberly-Clark and Procter & Gamble, to dominate the growing, adult incontinence market. Although their television commercials can be annoying, there is little doubt that this competition has brought about development of less bulky products offering improved absorbency, better comfort, and other desirable features.

Artificial Sphincters

Artificial urinary sphincters are a bagel-shaped prostheses designed to be surgically implanted in incontinent men or women. Once in place, this device surrounds the urethra in the same general area as the natural sphincter. A quantity of hydraulic fluid in the prosthesis applies continuous inward pressure on the urethra, choking off urine flow from the bladder.

In incontinent men, a small bulb is hidden within the scrotum. The fluid in the prosthesis is connected to the bulb through a narrow tube. When a man has an urge to urinate, he merely squeezes his scrotum in the vicinity of the bulb, which releases pressure inside the artificial sphincter and permits urine to flow from the bladder. A few minutes after voiding, fluid pressure within the prosthesis returns automatically to its normal level, once again preventing urine flow.

When performed by a competent urologist, artificial sphincter implantation is relatively simple and usually successful. When performed in a hospital, the procedure involves only a two- or three-day stay. Under appropriate anesthesia, the operation is painless and involves minimal surgical risk. A very small number of patients may experience some minor postoperative discomfort and possibly some treatable local infection. Depending on your location, the medical facility you select, and related factors, the procedure can cost less than $10,000, and should be covered by most insurance policies.

Artificial sphincters are made from the same inert, silicone plastic materials and are usually manufactured by the same companies as the penile implants discussed in Chapter 7. Safety concerns about female silicone breast implants have not been raised with either artificial sphincters or penile implants because silicone-containing fluids in breast implants are not used with either of these devices.

An artificial sphincter implantation is highly suitable for a broad spectrum of patients. I have men patients in whom I have successfully installed both artificial urinary sphincters and penile implants. Adequate room exists within the body for both devices and even then, there is little visual evidence of their presence nor do they represent a major obstacle to normal physical activities.

Catheters

In effect, a urinary catheter is a tube that for men is inserted through the tip of the penis into the urethra. The best known is the Foley, a device often employed with hospital patients recovering from surgery. The tip of the Foley is inserted until it enters the bladder. A small bulb at the tip, when inflated, holds the tube in place. Once it's secure, urine flows continuously into a concealed leg bag or some other container.

However, extended use of a Foley catheter can cause unpleasant irritation at the tip of the penis. The device can also cause urinary tract infections and bladder stones, so it is generally recommended only under continuing medical supervision. Most interest nowadays centers around intermittent catheters, which are inserted only from time to time. Typically, these devices are removed and reinserted every four hours or so.

Intermittent catheters are especially common in patients with spinal cord injuries. For postsurgery prostate patients, intermittent catheter use is well accepted. Many men are easily capable on their own of learning to manage this removal and reinsertion process. In men where age, physical condition, or sensitivity is a problem, these devices are generally inappropriate.

Drugs

Drugs for treating incontinence are in their infancy. Those investigated are meant to cause either increased constriction at the bladder outlet into the urethra or to prevent excess contractions higher up in the bladder. Antihistamines, for example, can improve muscle tone at the neck of the bladder, which is why men with incontinence sometimes notice an improvement when they take over-the-counter antihistamines for the relief of common colds or allergies.

Other drugs that have been tested include the antidepressant impramine and propantheline bromide for treating peptic ulcers, sold under the name Pro-Banthine. Unfortunately, many of the drugs investigated so far have undesirable side effects. Antihistamines frequently cause dizziness and a degree of sedation, so they should be used cautiously in patients with asthma, cardiovascular problems, and other conditions. Impramine can cause cardiac problems, weakness and fatigue, allergic reactions, and other symptoms. Propantheline bromide is associated with cardiac problems and should also be avoided by glaucoma patients.

Generally, drugs for treating incontinence are not too effective when damage to the sphincter muscles from prostate surgery is severe. They may help where the damage is relatively minor or where other factors contribute to incontinence. But the pace of research in this area is accelerating and it is likely that more effective and safer drugs will eventually become available.

Some types of drugs can also cause incontinence. From time to time, patients should present a list of all the medications they are taking to their urologist, and have the doctor check to see if any problems might be caused by their medications. Several drugs prescribed for other conditions can affect continence, including alpha adrenergic antagonists, diuretics, antihistamines, tranquilizers, or others.

Kegel Exercises

Kegel or pubococcygeal exercises, dating to about 1950, were developed originally by Dr. Arnold H. Kegel, a gynecologist, who expected they would help women overcome episodes of incontinence after childbirth. Later, the same exercises were found to help incontinent men, too, including those who had prostate surgery.

Kegel exercises are performed by tensing and tightening the pubococcygeus muscle in the vicinity of the rectum. Even if its name is unfamiliar, you have been aware of it most of your life—this is the muscle you feel whenever you strain to start or stop your urine flow while voiding. You can learn to do the Kegel properly by using the muscle repeatedly to interrupt your urine flow. In time, you will no longer need to urinate by exercising the muscle and can even make your penis bob up and down without using your hands.

Quick Kegels consist of rapidly tightening and relaxing the muscle. In slow Kegels, the muscle is tightened to a count of five, then relaxed. Four sets of each exercise should be performed each day, with the number of Kegels per set gradually increased. For all you know, you may once have talked to someone who was quietly doing some Kegels, because the exercise can be performed without attracting attention whether standing or sitting. Positive results may take up to three months, but after that a Kegel or two immediately before getting up from a chair or hearing a great joke may help avert an accident.

Muscle training exercises may be valuable in limiting the duration of post prostate incontinence. They can frequently cure mild stress urinary incontinence, and can greatly improve moderate stress urinary incontinence. Do not wear a clamp, a condom catheter, or an incontinence bag when you are recovering from surgery or radiation, because these will not allow you to develop the muscle control you need to become continent.

There have been some claims that the Kegel also provides sexual performance benefits. Some women who practice the Kegel are said to enjoy greater pleasure during intercourse, along with their partners. Men who practice the Kegel are said to have better ejaculatory control. It is difficult to substantiate these claims, but there is no reason not to try them yourself.

Kegel exercise devices made of rubber-coated steel are also available for about $35. The device is designed to be held tightly in the crotch. By squeezing the device, more tension is presumably placed on the muscle than during a normal Kegel. However, most authorities don't believe the device is worth its cost.

External Collection Devices

Incontinent men have one obvious advantage over women when it comes to external collection devices. A typical device for men is made of soft rubber and resembles a condom, which is pulled over the penis and held in place by a band around the waist. A drainage tube connects the device to a collection bag secured to one of the user's legs by a band. An external collection device can also be used with a penile clamp to control urine flow.

External collection devices are a relatively inexpensive means for dealing with incontinence. However, many men find them uncomfortable and cumbersome. For some, there may also be a problem in achieving adequate physical connection between the penis and the device. I have corrected that problem in several cases with a semirigid penile implant (see Chapter 7). With the implant in place, there is adequate extension of the penis to produce a tight connection and the implant also provides a workable solution for simultaneous impotence problems.

To avoid infection, external collection users are cautioned to clean themselves frequently and to replace parts of the system regularly. Men who use a penile clamp with an external collection device are cautioned not to apply too much pressure because they might dangerously restrict blood flow through the penis. Some men swear by external collection devices, while others, for the reasons indicated above, swear at them.

Help for Incontinent People, whose toll-free number is listed in the back of this book, will provide a free sixty-page catalog entitled *Resource Guide of Continence Products and Services* that lists all types of American products for this purpose, cross-referenced with their manufacturers. Your nurse or continence advisor may be consulted to educate you as to the use of these products as well as skin care.

Injections

Collagen is a naturally occurring protein found in the connective tissues that make up the joints and the bones of animals, including humans. Common gelatine desserts are mainly flavored collagen.

Some incontinent men are helped when small quantities of highly purified collagen are injected into the neck of their bladders. Polytef, a synthetic substance based on silicone, has physical properties similar to collagen, and is sometimes used in this manner. A 1994 study in Cleveland, Ohio, utilized a cross-linked collagen, Contigen, and was completed with good results on many patients. Contigen is purified collagen derived from cows which was chemically linked with glutaraldehyde. Injected around the urethra or bladder neck area, collagen injections can increase a patient's ability to contain leakage. This procedure may be done under local anesthetic, without foreign-body reactions, but it does require a urologist with considerable experience to reach correct tissue depth during injection. Many patients in the Cleveland study achieved continence after initial injections, but some had to be reinjected due to the tendency of the material to degrade over time. You should discuss this alternative with your urologist. Injection is not suitable for some situations such as those which require the placement of an artificial urinary sphincter. Teflon is also being studied as a material to be used for this purpose.

Typically, a series of several injections is required before any improvement is noted. The procedure is simple, causes minimum discomfort, and is relatively inexpensive.

Reconstructive Surgery

Unfortunately, until recently, the results from reconstructive surgery to correct incontinence in men whose sphincter muscles were damaged by transurethral or radical prostatectomy have generally been discouraging. Research is still underway in this area and it is likely that with improvement in surgical techniques, an increasing number of men should be helped by this surgery.

At this stage, reconstructive surgery is limited to experimental procedures designed to strengthen and reinforce the sphincter muscles. No techniques yet exist to repair damage to the sphincter nerves. Ask your urologist whether reconstructive surgery offers any real promise in your case. If so, you will probably be referred to a specialist.

Other Approaches to Managing Incontinence

A number of approaches for managing incontinence have been tried with varying success, including electrostimulation, electrical implants, biofeedback, and behavioral therapy.

Electrostimulation

In electrostimulation, a mild electrical current promotes involuntary contractions of the sphincter. The shock does not cause serious discomfort. Electrostimulation is believed to improve the strength and tone of the sphincter muscles and to lower the incidence of involuntary bladder contractions. When treating men, an electrode is usually inserted through the rectum. Each treatment session consists of a series of electric shocks between brief rest intervals. Studies have shown up to a 50 percent improvement in some patients, although there is no conclusive evidence of that degree of effectiveness in men who are incontinent because of prostate treatment.

Normally, if a reduction of symptoms doesn't occur within four or five treatments, the therapy is stopped. Treatments are continued until improvement no longer occurs.

In the United Kingdom and in Sweden, electrostimulation is considered a low-cost treatment with few side effects which can be used for a short period of time in the clinic or for long-term therapy. It is similar to Kegel exercises, but it is done passively rather than actively by the patient.

Electrical Implants

Similar to electrostimulation are electrical implants, battery-powered electrodes surgically installed in the sphincter muscles or the walls of the bladder. Electrical implants are only at an early stage of development.

Biofeedback

Biofeedback involves continous electronic monitoring of sphincter muscle contractions. The frequency and intensity of the contractions are observed by the patient on a video screen and signaled to him by sounds or lights. The theory is that by interacting with the contraction signals, men may eventually achieve better sphincter control. Biofeedback usually involves up to two sessions a week. The technique has yielded encouraging results in treating high blood pressure, and in incontinence, some studies indicate improvement in up to 10 percent of patients.

Biofeedback has the advantage of being a noninvasive, low risk procedure and it can lead to significant improvement. Your physician or nurse may recommend a practitioner skilled in biofeedback. Another source of a clinician trained in this technique is the Association for Applied Psychophysiology and Biofeedback in Wheat Ridge, Colorado. However, it is doubtful biofeedback will prove to be much help in men with serious sphincter damage from prostate treatment.

Behavioral Therapy

Behavioral (or behavior) therapy is based on systematic psychological conditioning, involving a weekly series of lengthy and intensive sessions designed to retrain patients in bladder control. They are required to keep records of their voiding symptoms and these records are an important basis for each weekly session. Some studies show improvement in as many as 85 percent of cases. Behavioral therapy is expensive and has not been too effective in men who have had prostate treatment.

Keeping a Uro-log helps patients make themselves aware of their urinary habits. Patients who have had trouble with bladder control are sometimes asked to keep a record of their symptoms for a week prior to an appointment with their urologist. This helps the doctor clearly understand the symptoms, which are sometimes too numerous to remember in a short office visit.

Some studies have shown improvement or cure rates for incontinence from 47 to 100 percent with simple strategies of behavior modification, although this success depends on selecting patients who might be helped by this strategy. Behavior modification also requires frequent instruction and reinforcement by the medical team.

An educational strategy to modify behavior consists of three steps. The first step is to educate the patient about lower urinary function, using diagrams or models or whatever educational aids are useful. The second step is to establish a voiding schedule, have the patient keep a record of it, and to teach the patient to use deep breathing or muscle contraction techniques to stop the urge to urinate for a few minutes, or until the scheduled time. Gradually, with a lot of positive reinforcement, the times are lengthened until patients reach up to a three to four hour voiding interval. Positive reinforcement over the telephone and in person is crucial to success with this method.

Psychotherapy

Psychotherapy can be helpful in managing incontinence. Where patients have no physical cause for their incontinence, psychotherapy can help to reveal and treat emotional factors that may underlie the problem. With men incontinent after prostate treatment, psychotherapy may provide relief from the emotional burden associated with their condition. This can be particularly helpful for men whose emotional response to incontinence is influenced heavily by their toilet training.

There are many forms of psychotherapy, ranging from intensive traditional psychoanalysis to relatively simple counseling. Most tend to be expensive.

Environmental Factors

Environmental factors can contribute to incontinence. Making the toilet accessible and visible can help, as can removal of any physical barriers which can get in the way of the patient who must go to the bathroom. If a patient needs a walker or a cane to make his way to the toilet, those items should be close at hand. Handrails or other safety devices may be installed in the home, the bathroom, or the shower if needed.

If You Are Incontinent

If you become incontinent after prostate treatment, there are several things you can do to take personal control of the situation.

See Your Urologist

Your urologist's responsibility is not over after your initial recovery from prostate surgery. If postsurgical treatment for incontinence is not a specialty of your urologist, ask for a referral to a doctor who is a specialist.

In my practice, I encourage frequent follow-up visits after prostate surgery or radiotherapy, not only to evaluate the treatment program, but to provide solutions for treatment side effects such as incontinence and associated emotional problems. I have yet to encounter a male patient whose physical problems with incontinence could not be helped. I have also found that a simple office discussion usually deals effectively with the emotional impact of incontinence. I encourage my patients to talk freely about their early toilet training and about current attitudes on incontinence, such as their feelings toward incontinent persons. Then, I try to put the overall problem in a realistic perspective. Of course, some men may require more intensive counseling, due to their feelings of guilt and other deep-seated emotional attitudes.

Watch Your Diet

Poor diet can exacerbate incontinence. Too much food, along with insufficient exercise, leads to obesity, which increases pressure on the bladder. Often, only a modest reduction in body weight can considerably improve incontinence. Constipation also contributes to incontinence, and the best answer to that is a healthy diet rich in bulk and fiber, NOT a laxative. Some excellent foods include most fruits and leafy vegetables, whole-grain bread, bran cereals, beans, and lentils.

A diuretic is any food or drug that promotes urination. Foods that are diuretic should be eaten in moderation because they will make your incontinence worse. They include coffee, tea, soft drinks containing caffeine, and alcohol. Grapefruit and grapefruit juice also have a diuretic effect. Diuretic drugs are prescribed often for individuals with high blood pressure and tissue swelling (edema). Don't stop taking necessary drugs like these without consulting your physician. Especially in cases of high blood pressure, it is possible to substitute an effective drug that has no diuretic effect.

Many people have reported to Help for Incontinent People that bladder symptoms including urgency, frequency, and increased leakage have come directly from caffeinated beverages, carbonated beverages, highly spiced foods, citrus juice and citrus fruits, alcohol, decaffeinated coffee, chocolate, and sugar. A few people have had trouble with aspartame.

Try eliminating one or more of the following items and see if it helps: alcoholic beverages, beer, wine, colas, coffee, tea, milk or milk products, corn syrup, citrus drinks or fruits, medicines containing caffeine, sugar, honey, chocolate, tomatoes, tomato-based products, and highly-spiced foods.

Cranberry juice, grape juice, cherry juice, and apple juice are thirst-quenching beverages which do not bother the bladder. Cranberry and cherry juice also help control odor. The best beverage of all is water—perhaps with a very thin slice of lemon to improve the taste.

Other factors which can contribute to incontinence include excess weight, since obesity puts a strain on the bladder. Groups such as Overeaters' Anonymous or Weight Watchers are simple, inexpensive programs which have helped many people lose weight. And if you can, stop smoking, too, since tobacco smoke irritates the bladder and may cause leakage.

Schedule Your Fluid Intake

Always drink plenty of water. You can schedule to your best advantage those times during the day when you drink water, and avoid drinking water and other fluids beyond your normal needs.

Given the problem of sleeping through the night, it is a good idea to limit fluid intake following your evening meal to no more than one cup. During the day, two or three quarts will generally provide adequate fluid intake. Of course, you should drink more when you exercise heavily or are subjected to dehydrating temperatures and humidity.

Some incontinent individuals severely limit their fluid intake in the mistaken belief it will help their condition. Too little water not only results in dark-colored urine, but can also worsen an incontinence problem and result in constipation. It is also unhealthy and potentially dangerous in the elderly if the daily intake of water falls below one and a half quarts.

Making the toilet facilities as convenient as possible will help. Bedside commodes are available, as are bedpans or urinal pads which may be placed on the bed and replaced. Clothes which are easy to get on and off are recommended. To prevent accidents, many men are advised to use the toilet when they first notice the urge to void, rather than forcing themselves to wait. Do not hurry the patient— allow him to remain on the toilet until he feels his bladder or bowels are empty.

Practice Good Hygiene

If you are incontinent, careful hygiene is essential. Failure to clean the areas of your body exposed to urine often results in uncomfortable and sometimes serious skin irritations and infections. Frequent cleaning with plain soap and water followed by application of a moisturing cream will usually protect the skin and avoid odor.

The newer, disposable absorbent products on the market have simplified this problem. Disposable wipes are also available that make things easier away from home. Avoid any products containing deodorizers that might cause allergic reactions.

Do Not Withdraw from Society or Give Up on Sex

Unfortunately, many individuals react to incontinence by avoiding all social contacts, which not only affects their quality of life, but can create an obvious problem for most of us who have to work for a living. With a positive attitude and some degree of persistence, almost any individual can come up with a system that permits normal social activities, including a job and even vigorous exercise.

If you are incontinent, there is no reason to give up sex either. Still, many individuals avoid sex, fearing an embarrassing accident. Precautions can be as simple as limiting fluid intake for about an hour before sexual activity and voiding immediately before. Bedding can be protected by towels and water-repellent sheets. It is even possible for a man with an internal catheter in place to experience rewarding sex. To do so, fold the catheter backward on your penis, put on a condom, and tape it in place. The condom and your partner's vagina should be well-lubricated with a water-soluble lubricant, not an oil-based product like petroleum jelly.

Infertility and the Prostate

Male infertility makes it impossible to father children. It can have two possible causes: any condition that prevents seminal fluid from reaching the unfertilized egg within the body of the female partner; some defect in the quality of the seminal fluid and the sperm it contains.

Prostate problems can contribute to infertility in both ways. When retrograde ejaculation follows prostate surgery, infertility results, because the seminal fluid cannot travel the normal route into the female partner. Retrograde ejaculation and incontinence are related; both conditions result from surgical damage to the same part of the body. Prostatitis can also cause infertility by creating defects in the seminal fluid and in the sperm.

Retrograde Ejaculation

In retrograde ejaculation, the same sphincter muscle involved in incontinence fails to function properly during sexual intercourse. Normally, the sphincter tightly closes the passageway through which urine travels from the bladder. When it does, semen travels down through the penis. When a sphincter is damaged and retrograde ejaculation results, the semen follows the line of least resistance and flows into the bladder, not the penis. Unfortunately, there is usually enough damage to the sphincter during any type of prostatectomy to cause retrograde ejaculation. Greater damage can cause incontinence, too.

A man with retrograde ejaculation can experience normal orgasm, so it is not always readily apparent to him that the condition exists. Sometimes, the first clue is slightly cloudy urine in the toilet bowl when you void for the first time after ejaculation. The only true test, however, is absence of seminal fluid after masturbation. But don't ever count on retrograde ejaculation for birth control, because the condition does not always result in *all* the semen backing up in the bladder.

Most men who experience retrograde ejaculation are at an age and in a family situation where fertility is no longer a concern. But there can be exceptions, such as Wolf, fifty, a retired oil tanker captain, who avoided marriage during his twenty-five-year career in the merchant marines. He felt very strongly that his long absences at sea would harm a family relationship. Shortly after retirement and a marriage to a women twenty years his junior, the need for prompt surgical treatment for BPH became apparent. When discussing the procedure, I informed Wolf about the high likelihood of retrograde ejaculation and its consequences for fertility. Before the operation, at my suggestion, Wolf arranged to store some of his sperm in a local sperm bank. Later, with that sperm, the couple became parents.

Fortunately, a solution still exists even for men who failed to bank their sperm before surgery and who still desire children:

1. Ejaculate either by intercourse or masturbation.
2. Immediately after ejaculation, urinate into a container.
3. Take the filled container to a gynecologist's laboratory and have the sperm recovered by filtration.
4. The female partner is artificially inseminated with the recovered sperm.

An alternative is to draw sperm from your bladder through a catheter. The brief exposure of the sperm to your urine will not affect their potency or result in birth defects.

I always ask any man before prostate surgery whether future children will ever be desired, even when a negative answer seems obvious to me. I also mention sperm storage, realizing some men are unsure about their future intentions. Sperm storage can be a wise precaution. An interesting example is provided by a patient who recently fathered a child at fourty-four by artificial insemination. Twelve years earlier, before he even married, he took the precaution of storing sperm before a necessary orchiectomy for testicular cancer.

Prostatitis and Infertility

The full story of how prostatitis causes male infertility is still unknown and the subject is a medical controversy. Reasonable clinical evidence exists that certain organisms associated with prostatitis can adversely affect both the physical structure and the motility (movement) of sperm. In some men suffering from prostatitis, sperm have been observed with abnormalities such as two heads or two tails or even no tails. With poor motility, sperm can't make it to their goal.

Microorganisms linked to male infertility include e. coli, the most common cause of bacterial prostatitis. E. coli appears to affect both sperm structure and motility. Trichomonas vaginalis (trick) has also been identified as a possible cause of male infertility. Of course, it is true that many men who have been infected by these organisms have successfully fathered children, but the reasons why some become infertile and others do not are still unknown. Perhaps some men's sperm are more resistant than others or these infectious organisms have a greater effect on men whose sperm were impaired by other factors.

There are still many uncertainties, but there is general agreement that when an infertility problem appears to exist in a marriage, it is important to test the male partner for prostatitis and, if it is found, to treat the condition aggressively. If a condition like trick, which can be passed back and forth between partners, is found, both should be treated.

Despite continuing improvement in treatment techniques, permanent incontinence is sometimes an unavoidable consequence of prostate surgery and radiation therapy. An incontinent man has a wide range of options available for dealing with the problem. With these available solutions, there is no reason for an incontinent man not to live a productive and fully satisfactory life, or to avoid social activities or sex.

For some men, absorbent products are an effective solution. For others, artificial urinary sphincter implants can be very satisfactory. New ways to deal with incontinence are under development that may provide even better solutions in the future.

Infertility is principally a concern of younger men, although there can be exceptions. Prostate treatment can cause infertility when damage to urinary sphincter muscles results in retrograde ejaculation. Men awaiting prostate treatment who may want to father children, or who are in any doubt, should store some sperm in a sperm bank. Even when that is not done, an effective procedure exists for a man with retrograde ejaculation, enabling him to obtain a supply of sperm to artificially inseminate his partner. Prostatitis can also affect infertility, so its treatment is important enough in its own right, and may help some men overcome infertility.

The following chapter covers early warnings of prostate problems and tells you when to seek professional help. Early detection is vital, so the next chapter could be the most important in this book.

CHAPTER 9

Do I Have a Prostate Problem?

Greg hadn't felt quite right for several weeks. One day while urinating, the young man noticed a slight burning sensation. In time, the sensation became increasingly intense. Soon Greg began to notice a constant dull aching on the underside of his penis.

A close friend suggested that Greg should see a urologist. The problem was quickly identified: an easily treatable prostate infection.

Mel noticed he was wetting his underwear after urinating. He tried to be more careful, but to no avail. His wife pointed out that the forty-five-year-old computer programmer was getting up four or five times a night to go to the bathroom. She was worried, because frequent urination is a diabetes symptom.

After some urging on her part, Mel made a rare visit to his physician, a specialist in family practice. After examination, he was referred to a urologist, where BPH, an enlarged prostate, was confirmed and a suitable treatment program was begun.

Arnold, on the other hand, never had any symptoms. But he was lucky. A slight bump on the surface of his prostate was discovered during his routine annual physical. Fortunately, his prostate cancer was detected early, greatly improving his chances for successful treatment.

Prostate Symptoms

As Arnold's case demonstrates, there is no substitute for an annual examination of the prostate by a physician. However, there is an important role for self-diagnosis, too. The symptoms checklist in this chapter will help readers detect many prostate problems. The list is based on questionnaire data I request from all my new patients. The description of these symptoms indicates the importance of seeking professional medical advice.

When You Have Pain or Discomfort

Pain is your body's early warning system. Pain in the region of your prostate will often alert you to a prostate problem.

A burning sensation when you urinate can indicate prostate infection. Typically, the sensation is felt in the center of the penis along the urethra, the channel that carries urine and seminal fluid. Sometimes with infection, a dull, less intense pain can be felt on the underside of the penis, especially where the penis protrudes from the body. If that pain persists more than a few days, you should see a doctor.

Pain in the lower back or the groin can be associated with a prostate difficulty. It may also indicate a variety of other disorders, including back trouble and kidney and bladder problems. If your pain is intense or persists beyond a few days, visit a doctor.

An indication of prostate infection is pain felt during sexual intercourse, both before and during ejaculation. If a man experiences this pain often, he may avoid intercourse, a factor worth considering by the female partner. If painful intercourse persists, medical attention is suggested.

Finally, a general feeling of fatigue and malaise—sometimes with a low-grade fever—often accompanies prostate infections. Obviously, such symptoms are present in a variety of other illnesses, too. But a combination of fatigue and malaise with other symptoms such as painful urination suggests a possible prostate problem and indicates the need for medical treatment.

Symptoms You Can See

There are several symptoms you can see that signal prostate disorders or a similar condition. All are warnings to seek prompt medical attention.

A drip from the penis could be caused by a prostate infection or by some other malady, including a sexually transmitted disease. Blood in your urine should never be ignored. Call your doctor at once. The causes can range from simple prostate infections to cancer of the prostate, bladder, or kidney. Incidentally, that advice applies equally to women. Sometimes it is difficult to tell if blood is present simply by examining the contents of the toilet bowl after urinating. If you think there's blood in your urine, collect a sample in a jar and hold it up to the light. Especially dark, cola-colored urine may not have any blood present, because this appearance usually indicates a liver disorder. This symptom should also send you quickly to your doctor.

Blood in your seminal fluid is an almost sure sign of infection. To ascertain if blood is present, examine a sample of semen you collect in a condom during intercourse or masturbation.

Symptoms Involving Sexual Performance

Commonly, premature ejaculation occurs before vaginal penetration or very shortly thereafter. Most premature ejaculation is caused by a prostate infection, not a psychological factor. If you ejaculate prematurely, consult a urologist before you consider psychotherapy.

Men who experience premature ejaculation or pain during sex often avoid intercourse altogether. The partners of these men would be wise to bring up these issues. A highly variable pattern of sexual intercourse, as with men who travel for long periods, can be a factor in prostate irritation that will be considered by your urologist should you have prostate irritation, but no evidence of infection.

Voiding Symptoms

The voiding patterns discussed in this chapter are helpful in determining if a man has prostate enlargement. Men who suffer from an extreme urgency to urinate often have enlarged prostates, which does not mean that a young man who has drunk too much beer at a Fourth of July picnic and is unable to find a convenient rest facility is a candidate for prostate treatment.

An inability to initiate urine quickly, straining to pass urine, and a weak and intermittent urinary stream are all signals of prostate enlargement. If the bladder fails to empty completely, that is another sign. One or more episodes of total retention offer absolute evidence. Total retention is a potentially fatal and painful medical problem demanding an immediate trip to a hospital emergency room. All retention episodes should have follow-up treatment by a urologist in order to identify the underlying cause.

Wetting yourself before or after urinating should be viewed in proper perspective. All mothers are familiar with the five year old so wrapped up in play that he has an accident. Back in our university days, a time when prostate enlargement is rare, we first heard the old couplet, "No matter how much you dance or prance, that last drop goes down your pants." However, in older men a pattern of wetting, which can be gauged by size and frequency of underwear stains, indicates a prostate enlargement problem.

Frequent urination, especially at night, should always be investigated promptly. Any healthy male should be able to sleep through the night without urinating, or with no more than a single trip to the bathroom. If urination becomes more frequent, see a doctor.

Incontinence, the accidental loss of urine, also calls for a visit to your urologist. Individuals who had bedwetting problems during their late childhood years are more prone as adults to suffer from a condition known as medium-bar obstruction, a blockage at the neck of the bladder. Men with medium-bar obstruction find urination difficult. The condition should not be confused with urinary problems caused by prostate enlargement.

Test Kits

A typical urine test kit contains paper strips, a color-coded comparison chart, and instructions. Ask your physician to provide you with a supply of strips for home testing.

You simply dip a test strip in your urine sample and compare the resulting color against the kit chart. One strip in each kit detects blood in the urine. This strip can detect blood at levels that cannot be seen by the human eye or when the urine is off-color from other causes. A second strip detects unusually large numbers of white blood cells, which accumulate in urine if the body's immune system is fighting an infection.

Getting Help

Many individuals with prostate problems see their own physician first. Typically a specialist in family practice or internal medicine, your personal physician will usually refer you to a urologist. This referral by a designated "primary care provider," or so-called "gate keeper," is usually mandatory in managed-care health programs such as HMOs.

Too many Americans have no regular relationship with a physician. If you're one of them, and you think you have a prostate problem, consult a urologist on your own. Contact your local medical society for the name of a conveniently located urologist. The society will usually provide a list of names from which you can make your selection. You can also write or call the American Urological Association, 1120 North Charles Street, Baltimore, MD 21201 (telephone (301) 727-1100). On your first visit to a urologist, take along a written copy of your answers to the checklist on the next page.

Urologists specialize in the urinary systems in both men and women. For men, urologists also treat genital problems, including prostate disorders, male infertility, and sexual dysfunction, including impotence and premature ejaculation. Urologists also perform vasectomies when infertility is desired for family planning, as well as vasectomy reversals, when patients wish to restore their fertility.

Because so many urologists handle "male problems," they are being referred to increasingly as the "male doctor," someone to turn to for advice and treatment in this area. Their role with men parallels gynecologists, who specialize in "female problems."

Except in clear emergencies, such as blood in your urine and urine retention, most of you have some latitude in arranging medical appointments, so you can reasonably delay a visit until you have significant evidence. Remember one vital point: Home diagnosis is NEVER a substitute for an annual physical examination that includes a digital rectal examination of your prostate.

PROSTATE SYMPTOM CHECKLIST

Symptoms of Pain or Discomfort

Do you experience a burning sensation
while urinating?   Yes____   No____

Do you ever notice a dull aching on the
underside of your penis?   Yes____   No____

Are you experiencing low back pain or
pain in the groin area?   Yes____   No____

Do you ever experience pain during sexual
intercourse, either before or during ejaculation?   Yes____   No____

Have you recently been feeling tired or
generally run down?   Yes____   No____

Symptoms You Can See

Is there any drip from your penis?   Yes____   No____

Is there any sign of blood in your urine?   Yes____   No____

Does your urine seem exceptionally cloudy or syrupy? Yes____   No____

Symptoms Involving Sexual Performance

After sex, have you noticed blood in your ejaculate? Yes____   No____

Do you often experience premature ejaculation?   Yes____   No____

Have you recently been avoiding sexual intercourse?   Yes____   No____

Is your frequency of sexual intercourse highly
variable due to the availability of a partner?   Yes____   No____

Voiding Symptoms

Describe the "urge" you usually feel before urinating.　None____
　Mild____
　Moderate____
　Severe____

Do you begin to urinate as soon as you want to?　Yes____　No____

Do you ever strain or force yourself to pass urine?　Yes____　No____

Describe the force of your urinary stream.　Normal____
　Variable____
　Weak____
　Dribbling____

Is your stream continuous or does it slow down
or even stop halfway through urination?　Continuous____
　Intermittent____

Do you feel that your bladder empties completely?　Yes____
　Sometimes____
　Not usually____

Do you ever wet yourself before or after urinating?　Yes____　No____

How many times do you urinate at night?　0 to 1____
　2____
　3 to 4____
　More____

How often do you urinate during the day?　Every three hours
　or more____
　Every 1 to 2 hours____
　Every 2 to 3 hours____
　Every hour____

At what age did you stop bedwetting?　____

Do you ever experience urinary incontinence
(accidentally losing urine)?　Yes____　No____

CHAPTER 10

Exercise and Your Prostate

Almost every part of your body benefits from regular exercise and your prostate is no exception. Two types of exercises can help keep your prostate healthy. The first promotes overall physical fitness, which helps your prostate only indirectly, but does so in a number of crucial ways. The second type is specific to the prostate and nearby organs in the pelvic area.

General Physical Fitness— Benefits and Suggestions

Cliff, mentioned in Chapter 6, who had a radical prostatectomy for prostate cancer, was in and out of the hospital in a few days. His excellent physical condition made him a fine candidate for surgery. Despite the nuisance of a Foley catheter, Cliff was on his feet and walking a few hours after the operation. He returned to work and resumed all his normal physical activities in well under the usual six to eight weeks usually needed for full recovery after a prostatectomy.

When he was asked why he struggled to keep in shape, Cliff's explanation had always been "you never know when your car might break down in the middle of nowhere and you'll have to walk miles to get help." Regular exercise paid off for Cliff, as it will for everyone.

Breezing through a prostate operation with a minimum of complications is only one of the ways your prostate will be helped by a conscientious fitness program. Regular exercise can also help your prostate by:

- Lowering your cholesterol—Exercise reduces LDL, the so-called "bad cholesterol" and elevates HDL, the "good cholesterol." There is evidence cholesterol may be a factor in prostate enlargement.
- Preventing obesity—Layers of excess body fat around the prostate place a strain on the gland and surrounding tissues and may contribute to voiding problems. Along with poor muscle tone in your lower body, obesity can also contribute to lower back pain and is sometimes a factor in prostatodynia.
- Improving cardiovascular fitness—Exercise improves circulation, raises blood oxygen levels, and improves oxygen utilization. The prostate benefits from increased blood flow and the improved quality of blood that reaches the gland.

Appropriate General Fitness Programs

A physical fitness program appropriate for you depends on your age and general condition. Unfortunately, the many young men who engage in active sports, work out vigorously in health clubs, or jog are a distinct minority of the total adult male population. Most men get their "exercise" watching sports on television and don't usually break that pattern until sometime in their late thirties or early forties, and only after being scolded by a worried physician. By then, some are also reaching a point when symptoms of benign prostate enlargement may appear.

Exercise involving a combination of prolonged sitting and jarring, repeated motions such as riding a horse or motorcycle can stress the prostate. This may be a reason why farmers, as a group, have a disproportionately high rate of prostate cancer because their prostate glands are frequently jarred by activities such as driving a tractor or combine.

If you have engaged in regular, strenuous physical activity such as tennis, jogging, and skiing, there should normally be no reason to change that pattern when you reach your late thirties and early forties. However, for most men approaching their prostate problem years, swimming or walking are usually more appropriate exercises. Low-impact aerobics is a good choice, too.

A study of 17,000 Harvard graduates published in 1992 showed that men who exercised frequently had much lower rates of prostate cancer than men who were sedentary. Another study of women at the University of Southern California showed that high rates of exercise helped prevent breast cancer, which, like prostate cancer, is a hormone-dependent cancer.

Swimming

Swimming gives you an excellent cardiovascular workout and is good exercise for most muscles, including those in the pelvic area. Benefits from swimming are derived with virtually no pain and there is little danger of injuring your joints, muscles, or skeletal structure, owing to the cushioning effect of water. Swimming is also fun and helps to relieve emotional frustrations.

A daily thirty-minute swim is recommended, although some benefits can be obtained when you swim as few as three times a week. Ideally, you should put enough effort into your swimming to elevate your heart rate to an optimum level appropriate for your age and condition. You don't have to devote your entire workout to frantic, boring "laps."

Absent of any special health problems, most men should not be overly stressed by a thirty-minute swim. However, there are a few precautions. If you have chronic prostatitis, avoid swimming in cold water (75° F or below), or you may trigger an acute attack. Always get your urologist's permission before swimming if you are recovering from prostate surgery. Swimming really aids surgery recovery, especially after abdominal surgery, but you are risking infection if you swim before your incision has healed.

Walking and Hiking

Walking is excellent both for the entire body and for the mind. By contrast with jogging, you have more time to think and to enjoy the scenery. Unlike jogging, there is no risk of joint damage.

For best results, walk at least two miles a day at a brisk pace, stopping only briefly and occasionally. A few modest hills will add to the value of your walk. There is nothing wrong with "power walking," using hand weights, although that tends to turn a generally pleasurable experience into more of a chore.

Walking is usually safe and appropriate for men with prostate problems. However, men with benign prostate enlargement, who often experience a sudden and urgent need to void, may have a practical problem. Always wear proper shoes and take extra care in high temperatures and humidity.

Hiking is good, too. Hikes of ten to fifteen miles a day, and even more, are not beyond the capability of most men in the prostate problem years. Cross-country skiing is a pleasant alternative to hiking.

A final word on walking: try skipping the elevator or escalator and walk up stairs. If you live close enough, why not walk to and from work?

Aerobics

Aerobic exercises are designed to improve cardiovascular fitness by elevating your heart and breathing rates for an extended period. Typically, aerobics sessions incorporate stretching to improve muscle flexibility. You can perform aerobics at home, but classes offer the benefits of a trained instructor and are less boring.

Aerobics can be low- and high-impact. Both provide equal benefits, but the low-impact exercises are easier on the joints and are generally more appropriate for older men. You will gain significant benefits from as few as three one-hour aerobics sessions a week. Depending on your overall health, most men with prostate problems will not find these sessions too stressful.

Water aerobics, also called aquaerobics or hydroaerobics, are an interesting alternative to conventional aerobics, providing all the usual benefits, but the exercises are usually easier to perform under water and for many men are more fun.

Prostate-Specific Exercises

Exercises of specific value to your prostate are those that enhance the suppleness and flexibility of muscles in the prostate area and promote improved blood flow to the gland and surrounding tissues. Appropriate prostate exercises include stretching, abdominal muscle control, and relaxing pelvic muscles. Exercises that contain some of these elements are often found in stretching exercises performed toward the end of a standard aerobics workout.

Following are some prostate-specific exercises (in order of importance) you can easily perform at home.

Pelvic Thrusts

A simple exercise that really helps improve muscle tone in the prostate area is the pelvic thrust. This can be performed while seated by simultaneously squeezing your buttocks, pulling in on your lower abdominal and anal areas, and thrusting your pelvis forward. Each thrust should be held for several seconds, followed by a few seconds of relaxation. About ten thrusts should be performed in each exercise cycle. Do three or four cycles a day and even more when traveling.

Seated pelvic thrusts are good for men whose occupations require frequent long-distance trips in vehicles or airplanes. You can do the exercise while driving, but don't let it interfere with control of your vehicle. Pelvic thrusts are a standard routine in water aerobics classes for both men and women.

Kegel Variations

The Kegel exercises in Chapter 8 can help control urinary incontinence by strengthening the pubococcygeous muscle near the rectum. Variations on the Kegel can also improve muscle tone in the prostate area.

In one variation, sit crosslegged. After relaxing, pull your anal area inward as if you were trying to postpone a bowel movement. Hold that position for about ten seconds, then relax. About ten inward pulls and periods of relaxation constitute an exercise cycle.

Another variation is done with your knees and elbows on the floor, your legs bent at the knee, and your buttocks extending upward. From that position, contract your lower abdominal and anus muscles. Don't move your pelvis. This exercise relaxes the pelvis and back and helps men who complain of prostate-related back pain.

In a final Kegel variation, try consciously to flex your penis upward using only the muscles in the penile and rectal areas. You can do this exercise while either sitting or standing. Once mastered, you should be able to move your penis by as much as a half inch.

Abdominal Control Exercises

Abdominal control exercises strengthen abdominal muscles, flattening the abdomen and holding your abdominal muscles in place and with them your internal organs, including the prostate. They also strengthen the lower back and may help alleviate some prostatodynia symptoms. Old fashioned situps, like those done by generations of military recruits, are counterproductive, because they do not flatten the abdomen and may actually cause lower back pain.

The easiset abdominal control exercise is done standing with your feet slightly apart and your knees relaxed (never lock your knees). Put both hands together behind your head as if you were holding a sledge hammer to smash rocks. Rapidly move your hands forward and stop abruptly when they are above your head. Then relax. Performed properly, you will feel a sharp contraction in your lower abdomen. Repeat at least ten times.

Two abdominal control exercises can be done while seated. In the first, sit in a chair with your knees apart, and your head and shoulders partially bent. Keep your entire back snug against the chair. Do a series of at least ten outward and inward abdominal contractions, pausing to relax briefly between each one.

A variation on this exercise is to bend forward while sitting in a chair until both your outstretched hands, palms down, touch the floor, or come as close to the floor as you can get them. While in that position, repeat the previous series of abdominal contractions. This exercise relaxes and strengthens the lower back as well as the lower abdominal muscles.

Abdominal crunches or rollups are done lying on your back. In the simplest, spread your legs slightly, knees bent, with your hands held loosely together behind your head. Slowly raise your head and shoulders until the back of your head is about six inches above the surface, and hold it briefly. Then slowly lower your head and shoulders to the horizontal position. Repeat about ten times. You must elevate your head and shoulders using only your abdominal muscles. Never pull your head upward with your hands.

In a variation of the abdominal crunch, rotate your right arm and shoulder toward your left knee while slowly rising up as before, then alternate with your left arm and shoulder toward your right knee. You can also pause momentarily at intermediate positions during the full movements, holding your head and shoulders in place by flexing your lower abdominal muscles.

Reverse trunk rotations are done on your back, too. Lie flat, arms extended from your sides, knees bent. Extend your legs as far upward as you can and rotate to one side. Complete the movement when your legs touch the floor to one side. Then return to the original position and rotate to the opposite side. Repeat the rotations at least ten times on each side.

Squats

Slowly lower yourself to a sitting position, buttocks down, knees upward, with your hands or arms resting on your knees. Slowly rise to your original standing position. Repeat about ten times. To perform squats properly, both feet, including your heels, should rest entirely on the floor. It may take some practice before you can achieve the correct position, because the tendency is to balance on your toes with your heels several inches off the ground. As a variation, try moving about while maintaining the squat.

Squats will improve the muscle tone in your lower pelvic area. Throughout much of the world, the squat is the poor man's chair. In the Far East, many men and women effortlessly assume the squat for hours while performing daily activities such as cooking, selling goods in the market, even doing manual labor. The squat is also used frequently in the Far East for defecation, which from this position is more effortless and more complete, and relieves pressure on nearby organs including the prostate.

When learning to squat properly, you need to develop good stretch in the muscles of your thighs and calves. Frequent stretching of these muscles is desirable as you age, because that helps preserve flexibility and prevents loss of function. While learning the squat, it may help to hold onto a nearby sturdy object, like the railing dancers use when practicing classical ballet movement known as the plié, a partial knee bend, or semisquat performed standing with toes turned out and arms apart.

Other Exercises

Other exercises may also help the prostate. Sit on the floor, knees bent, your feet parallel and touching. Place a large, fairly rigid object between your knees, like a beachball or firm cushion. Then, tuck inward as far as you can with your knees and hold that position for about ten seconds. Relax for a few seconds and repeat. Pulling inward places pressure on your groin area and helps improve muscle tone.

Two others, cat stretches and pelvic lifts, may have some value to the prostate region. Cat stretches are done on your knees, facing down with your hands palms down on the floor supporting the front of your body. Arch your back and carefully and slowly stretch upward while exhaling. Hold the position for about three seconds while inhaling, then slowly relax to the original position. The cat stretch is principally a back exercise, but does provide some strengthening of the pelvic area.

Pelvic lifts are performed by lying on your back, knees bent upward, legs parallel, arms stretched out to the side. Lift your pelvic area as far as you can, supporting yourself and balancing with your lower back and feet. To do it properly, while in the upward position your body should form a straight line from your shoulders to your knees. Pelvic lifts are intended principally for the back and buttocks, but also have some positive effect in the pelvic area.

Yoga exercises may also offer positive benefits to the prostate. Yoga is a spiritual system based on Hindu ascetic and mystical philosophy that combines meditation with controlled breathing and certain physical postures called "asanas." Several asanas, such as the lotus, definitely help to stretch, relax, and improve muscle flexibility in the prostate area. Many people enjoy yoga.

Far too often in my practice I will encounter men who insist they can't exercise because of an existing prostate condition. That is no excuse not to maintain a healthy body weight and for keeping physically fit with an appropriate exercise program. The attitude is self-defeating, too, because proper exercise helps prevent and alleviate prostate problems.

Of course, before undertaking any program involving vigorous exercise, you should check with your physician, especially if you are out of shape or have a special problem, like a heart condition. Exercise *will* help your prostate.

The next chapter discusses diet, another important and closely related subject you can control that will help your prostate. Chapter 11 also contains advice on how to avoid so-called prostate "cures" that waste your money and may be harmful.

How to Promote
Your Own Prostate Health

Within a few years, the research now well underway in immunology, gene therapy, and other areas will produce far more effective treatments for prostate problems than those we've been discussing here. A new medical treatment may exist early in the next century that will prevent many prostate problems. Until then, there are plenty of things you can do now to improve your own prostate situation.

So far, you've already learned about suggestions for helping your prostate. Chapter 7 told you how to avoid prostate infections and how to assist in their cure. Chapter 8 made suggestions about sexual behavior that will help you avoid prostate irritation. Chapter 10 described useful prostate exercises.

This final chapter covers three other areas of prostate self help. The first addresses diet, nutrition, and beneficial drugs. The second takes a realistic look at the possible benefits of "alternative" medicine. The third tells how you and those close to you may be helped by the activities of a support group.

Diet, Nutrition, and Drugs

Scientific investigation has yet to develop any conclusive information on the relationship among prostate disorders, nutrition, and various drugs. This research is in its infancy, but should in time yield significant results. However, there are some areas where nutrition and certain drugs have been linked, at least preliminarily, to some aspect of prostate health:

- Obesity
- Diets promoting high levels of cholesterol
- Low levels of zinc in the prostate
- Vitamin intake
- Foods that irritate the prostate
- Drugs that irritate the prostate

Besides the above, certain diets and drugs can contribute to impotence and incontinence problems that may result unavoidably from prostate treatment, as discussed in Chapters 7 and 8. As yet, there is no evidence of a link between prostate disorders and important nutritional factors such as consumption of carbohydrates as either sugar or starch, or proteins. In proper quantities and in the correct forms, carbohydrates and proteins are vital to your overall health.

Every person should take into account the American Cancer Society's guidelines for good eating, which are carefully drawn to reduce the risk of cancer in all people. These seven general guidelines are:

1. Maintain a desirable body weight.
2. Eat a varied diet.
3. Include a variety of both vegetables and fruits in the daily diet.
4. Eat more high-fiber foods, such as whole-grain cereals, legumes, vegetables, and fruits.
5. Cut down on total fat intake.
6. Limit consumption of alcoholic beverages, if you drink at all.
7. Limit consumption of salt-cured, smoked, and nitrite-preserved foods.

Most health organizations now recommend that adults cut down the percentage of calories received from fat to about 30 percent of total intake, and eat at least five servings per day of fruits and vegetables, which contain no animal fat. Within the body, fat is chemically converted into androgens which stimulate the prostate. Average fat consumption in the United States is 37 to 40 percent of calories. Statistically, the risk of prostate cancer is higher for men who consume 40 to 60 percent of their total calories in the form of fat.

Studies comparing the diets of Americans and Europeans, who have a high rate of prostate cancer, and the diets of Asians, who have a low rate, show that men who eat high-fat diets have a much higher incidence of prostate cancer than do men who eat low-fat diets including yellow and green vegetables like carrots, cauliflower, and broccoli. When Asian men move to the United States and adopt an American diet, their levels of prostate cancer rise closer to the higher Caucasian American levels. The same variation in incidences of BPH are found when Asian and Caucasian American men are compared, with Asian men having many fewer instances of BPH.

Vitamin D, sometimes called the "sunshine vitamin," as well as sunlight itself seems to have some effect in inhibiting prostate cancer. Statistics show that men in the sunny Southern United States have lower rates of prostate cancer than do men in the less sunny North. Ultraviolet radiation on the skin is converted by the body into vitamin D. Fortified milk and fish are good dietary sources of vitamin D.

Several studies are currently underway, turning up good news regarding the prevention of cancer with food products made from soybeans. The Asian diet contains items made from soybeans such as soy sauce and tofu which may factor into their lower rates of BPH and prostate cancer. When mice are fed a diet high in soybeans, they have smaller prostate glands than mice on normal diets. Since prostate cancer is a hormone-dependent cancer, researchers speculate that consuming phytoestrogens like those in soybeans may benefit prostate health. Soybeans also contain other chemical elements believed to help stave off cancer such as protease inhibitors and phytoesterols.

All the antioxidant vitamins such as vitamin A, vitamin C, and vitamin E are believed to have a chemopreventive effect on cancer. Vitamin A, a fat soluble vitamin found in yellow vegetables like carrots, is an important part in the epithelial cells that line the prostate. In animal studies, vitamin A supplements have decreased prostate cancer although this has not been proven to help prostate cancer in human beings.

In the appendix, you'll find a week of menus that promote a healthy prostate. These menus incorporate what is now known about diet and the prostate. The appendix also includes suggestions on special diet problems caused by eating out.

Obesity

Obesity can cause physical strain on the prostate and the surrounding tissues in the lower abdominal area. A heavy accumulation of body fat in this region places pressure on all the organs crowded around the prostate and may contribute to a voiding problem caused by benign prostate enlargement. Obesity may also be a factor in prostate-related back pain and prostatodynia.

Obese patients are also at greater risk during prostate surgery for benign prostatic hyperplasia or prostate cancer and they have more problems recovering. Complications can arise during surgery because obese men are generally in poorer health than men with proper body weight. Layers of fat in an obese patient also make surgical procedures more complex. It takes obese men longer to get back on their feet and resume normal activities, which may mean a longer and more uncomfortable hospital stay and a longer recovery period at home.

To determine if you are obese, stand erect and squeeze a fold of skin on your abdomen just above your navel. If the fold is thicker than one inch, you are likely to be classed by your physician as obese, and advised to lose weight. The best way to do that is with a combination of a balanced diet and exercise, ideally under your physician's direction. It is not healthy to try to lose more than two pounds a week. To lose weight at that rate, you will have to increase daily physical activity and decrease daily caloric intake until you have a daily deficit of about 500 calories.

Long-term obesity control requires permanent adjustments to your level of physical activity and to your diet. Unfortunately, most men tend to put on weight as they age because they usually cut back on physical activities, failing to compensate by reducing daily calorie consumption. Adding to that problem is increased alcohol intake, which can add to your daily calorie load.

Diets That Promote
High Levels of Cholesterol

The belief that there may be a link between prostate tumors and cholesterol is based primarily on studies indicating that Asian men who eat a traditional diet have relatively low levels of both benign and malignant prostate tumors, while men of Asian extraction in the United States who eat a typical American diet experience tumors at about the same rate as other Americans. There is some reason to suspect a possible connection between prostate tumors and cholesterol because the hormone testosterone, known to promote tumor growth, has a chemical structure with important similarities to cholesterol. Thus, high levels of serum (blood) cholesterol may cause excess testosterone production.

However, experimental attempts to demonstrate such a link are inconclusive. In a Japanese study reported in 1989, rats fed a diet very high in cholesterol did not develop any tumors. Of course, there could be significant differences between what takes place in a rat prostate compared to a human prostate. Nevertheless, the findings with respect to prostate tumors in Asian men are sufficiently compelling to suggest that you should control your cholesterol in order to protect your prostate health. It is important to control your cholesterol anyway, in view of the well-established connection between high serum cholesterol levels and the higher-than-normal incidence of atherosclerosis. Besides, vascular problems that are often the result of too much cholesterol are among the factors implicated in many cases of impotence.

Cholesterol is produced naturally in your liver. A minimum cholesterol level in your blood is essential for production of certain hormones as well as the process that creates and sustains the cells in your nervous system. Your liver normally produces most of the cholesterol your body needs, but a certain amount is obtained from the foods you eat. Foods high in total fat, especially saturated fats, will increase your serum cholesterol level, possibly to a dangerous point.

To control your cholesterol and still enjoy tasty food, consider Asian cuisine. A typical meal consists of a mixture of chopped vegetables served over either a bed of rice, or wheat or rice noodles. Small quantities of meat added to the mixture are largely for seasoning and the meat is usually poultry or fish. When red meat is used, it is usually very lean. To stir fry the Asian meal, oils are used, not solid fats, with fish oils preferred. Typically, Asians also eat very few eggs or dairy products.

Asian meals require considerable preparation because the food is carefully chopped in advance so it can be eaten without a knife. You'll need to know something about spices, too. However, you can realize the health benefits of Asian cuisine without all that trouble if you simply eat a diet high in vegetables, fruits, and carbohydrates. Keep your total meat intake to a minimum and concentrate on fish and skinless poultry. Eat red meat only occasionally (perhaps as a reward on special occasions), and it should always be lean. Limit your intake of eggs, processed foods, and junk foods. Ideally, your diet should contain plenty of fiber and your carbohydrates should be mainly whole grains and coarse breads.

Any fat you use in cooking or add to your food should be polyunsaturated. These fats contain a large number of double bonds between the carbon atoms in their molecular structure. In saturated fats, hydrogen atoms fill the gaps between the carbon atoms. With the important exception of coconut and palm oil, oils provide more polyunsaturated fat than solid fats and shortenings.

It is important to be aware that *too little* cholesterol can also be a health problem owing to the essential need for cholesterol in human metabolism. Some medical researchers have suggested too-low cholesterol levels may even increase cancer risk, although not prostate cancer. That view, contrary to a widely held belief that individuals on diets high in fat, who typically have higher than normal levels of serum cholesterol, also are at increased risk for cancer. In a series of seventeen studies reviewed at a conference sponsored by the National Cancer Institute and the National Heart, Lung, and Blood Institute during the eighties, increased cancer risk was reportedly observed in individuals with cholesterol levels below 180. Cutting levels from 250 to 190, desirable in patients at risk of atherosclerosis, was *not* shown to increase cancer risks.

Now let's consider "good" and "bad" cholesterol. Good cholesterol is high-density lipoprotein or HDL; the higher its level in your overall cholesterol count, the fewer your chances of heart disease. However, the effect of the relative level of HDL on the prostate is not now known. Exercise definitely raises the level of HDL.

Low Levels of Zinc in the Prostate

For some time, zinc, a trace mineral, has been known to serve an important function in the prostate. What that is, however, is not yet clear. The prostate does contain a higher concentration of zinc than any other organ in the body; zinc is also present at high levels in semen. The mineral is recognized as important in human nutrition, and a recommended daily allowance (RDA) has been established by the National Research Council, Washington, D.C., the institution that establishes national nutrition standards.

Various theories have been suggested to explain zinc's role in the prostate, but none have yet been proved. One possibility is that the zinc has some effect on the activity of 5-alpha reductase. As discussed in Chapter 5, 5-alpha reductase, an enzyme found in the prostate, is involved in production of dihydrotestosterone

(DHT), the "bad" testosterone implicated in prostate tissue growth. Zinc may also be a factor on acid phosphatase levels and on the fertility of seminal fluid. Another theory suggests the prostate may even be the body's "warehouse" for zinc, releasing it when deficiencies develop in other parts of the body.

Severe zinc deficiency, rare in the United States but not in poor countries, has been linked to a variety of problems, including poor immune response, hair loss, skin rashes, poor growth, slow healing, and digestive problems. Some studies suggest low levels of zinc may be a factor in benign prostate enlargement. Because the mineral has some antibacterial activity, a zinc deficiency may lower your resistance to prostate infections.

Red meat, poultry, and seafood are excellent sources of dietary zinc. Typically, the American diet is high in these foods, the principal reason severe zinc deficiency has not been a problem in the United States. Some individuals who may be ingesting too little zinc may be experiencing mild to moderate zinc deficiency. Individuals particularly at risk include vegans and those on very low-calorie diets. A vegan is an extra-strict vegetarian who will not eat eggs, milk, cheese, any other dairy product, or animal flesh. Some other individuals have a problem absorbing zinc. Taking iron supplements, even when a component of multivitamin and multimineral supplements, has been found to lower zinc absorption in some people. Some studies also indicate that those who live in areas with hard water (of high total mineral content) also have lower levels of zinc in their systems.

I advise zinc supplements at moderate levels in men with prostate problems who have known zinc deficiencies, especially vegans. For others, given the current state of knowledge, it is still too early to suggest zinc supplements will benefit the prostate, although they won't hurt. Food consumed by all such men should, of course, always contain sufficient natural zinc.

While zinc supplements at moderate rates, 10 to 20 mg a day, are safe, megadoses at higher rates may not be. Some studies indicate that orally megadosing zinc does not always add any significant zinc to the prostate.

Be cautious about preparations containing zinc that are touted as impotence remedies. An advertisement for one such remedy, sold by mail, features a smiling gray-haired man embracing an obviously younger woman. As a specialist in impotence treatment, I assure you that such products are valueless, not to imply zinc does not have a beneficial effect on prostate health.

A Note on Magnesium

There are also suggestions that another trace mineral, magnesium, is of some relevance to the prostate. Magnesium deficiency has been linked to certain types of heart disease, and the mineral may also be a factor in transporting oxygen to the tissues, especially for those engaged in vigorous aerobic exercise. Low magnesium levels appear to be a factor in stone formation (calculi) in the urinary system, but no scientific studies have demonstrated any specific link to the prostate.

Many of the suggestions about magnesium's effect on the prostate originate from individuals in the hair-testing field. Hair testing is based on the belief that mineral deficiencies can be determined by analyzing a hair sample. However, this field is not held in high regard by the scientific community, although their ideas have influenced many patients.

You should get all the magnesium you need from a diet high in whole grains and leafy green vegetables. Magnesium supplements are not recommended, although available evidence indicates that doses at levels less than 300 mg a day are not harmful.

Vitamins and Prostate Health

Vitamins are complex organic chemical substances that have been proven by extensive scientific research to be *essential* in animal nutrition. With insufficient intake of any given vitamin, a serious nutritional disorder can be expected. To date, there is more reason to suspect a connection between prostate health and the vitamin A family (including beta carotene) and vitamins C and E.

Vitamin A and Beta Carotene

The vitamin A family includes vitamin A (in palmitate, acetate, propionate, and alcohol form) and beta carotene. Vitamin A, also known as retinol, is in the retinoid form. Beta carotene, also known as provitamin A, is in the carotenoid form.

Chemically, the carotenoid form is a dimer of the retinoid. Essentially, beta carotene is a heavy molecule in which two molecules of vitamin A are linked. When beta carotene is ingested, your liver converts each molecule of beta carotene into vitamin A.

Vitamin A is important in protecting good vision, in reproduction, and in tissue growth. In fact, "retinol" reflects the connection between vitamin A and the retina. An early symptom of vitamin A deficiency is night blindness. For some time, a vitamin A deficiency has been known to result in precancerous skin lesions. In 1975, positive evidence was presented in medical literature that both carotenoid and retinoid forms of vitamin A are useful in preventing and treating lung cancer. Major research efforts are underway under the auspices of the National Cancer Institute on the role of vitamin A in treatment of all major forms of cancer including prostate. Most of these efforts have centered around carotenoid vitamin A, not retinoid.

There is still no final proof that either beta carotene or vitamin A will help treat or prevent prostate cancer, but enough evidence is in for me to recommend that you should ingest daily an adequate quantity of vitamin A in either retinoid or carotenoid form. For an adult male, that means a total daily intake of 5,000 IU (International Units) from all sources each day.

In the retinoid form, Vitamin A is available naturally in whole milk, eggs, and animal products, especially liver. Beta carotene is present in a wide variety of fruits and vegetables. It is also the most common yellow coloring added to margarine, cheese, and other food products, which means you can get some vitamin A from those sources.

If you wish to take vitamin A supplements, I strongly recommend you take the vitamin in its beta carotene form. Beta carotene has been demonstrated to have far less toxicity than retinoid vitamin A, even in megadoses. Avoid large doses of retinoid vitamin A because of possible liver damage. Beta carotene also contains a larger number of unsaturated chemical double bonds than retinoid vitamin A. As a result, beta carotene is a better antioxidant, a property that helps to retard tissue aging.

Vitamin C

Known chemically as ascorbic acid, Vitamin C was found very early to play an important role in the treatment of the deficiency disease rickets. Recently, largely owing to the activities of Dr. Linus Pauling, there has been widespread interest in vitamin C as a treatment for the common cold. During the mid-seventies, Pauling began to publish papers suggesting a use for vitamin C in treating terminal cancer. In 1992, Pauling claimed vitamin C will shrink prostate tumors.

As a giant in the history of chemistry, Pauling's views cannot be dismissed casually. He is twice a Nobel laureate and his work on the chemical bond is the foundation of modern molecular theory. Conclusive experimental confirmation, however, does not yet support vitamin C as a treatment for prostate cancer. Nevertheless, vitamin C is generally considered nontoxic, with minimal side effects in most patients even at high dosage. Possible side effects are reported from megadoses of vitamin C, including gastritis and kidney problems.

Vitamin C is obtained naturally from most fruits and vegetables. My best recommendation is to increase your intake of vitamin C by eating more fruits and vegetables, especially citrus fruits. If you do take vitamin C supplements, it is best to avoid megadoses.

Vitamin E

Until recently, the full potential of vitamin E (tocopherol) has not been fully appreciated. An adequate supply of the vitamin has been found important in preventing degeneration of the muscle, nervous, and vascular systems. There is evidence that vitamin E specifically retards the aging process in reproductive tissues, which could include the prostate.

Vitamin E is known to be a highly effective intercellular antioxidant, which may explain why it helps prevent muscle degeneration. There is a known interrelationship between vitamin E and the mineral selenium in the complex chemical processes that take place within cells.

The RDA for vitamin E in adult males is 30 IU; and most men should be able to achieve that level through regular use of soybean, corn, sunflower seed, and rapeseed (canola) oils, and wheat germ, lettuce, and alfalfa. In these foods, the vitamin can be present at levels as high as 0.3 percent. If you are interested in vitamin E supplements, be aware that high dosage has been linked to elevated blood pressure. However, this vitamin is not considered toxic. I should also warn you that supplemental doses of selenium should be taken with caution. High concentrations of the mineral are quite toxic. Furthermore, elevated levels of selenium cause very bad breath.

Foods That Can Irritate the Prostate

The prostate has a peculiar property: It can trap many chemical substances taken into the body with foods you eat. These substances reach the prostate through the bloodstream. Once inside, it is difficult for them to get out, so they may remain for a long time and cause considerable irritation.

The principal foods and beverages that can cause prostate problems are those that are highly spiced or contain alcohol or caffeine. Typically, highly spiced foods contain quantities of cayenne (chili), tabasco, jalapeño, or other types of peppers. Peppers contain high levels of volatile oils—pungent, low-molecular weight, oily substances that easily evaporate. Due to their volatility, such oils have a special tendency to concentrate in the prostate, where the same properties of these oils that make you sneeze or cough when eating "hot" foods can also irritate the gland. That does not mean never again enjoying a meal at your favorite Thai or Mexican restaurant, but it does suggest avoiding a steady diet of such foods.

Alcohol is very readily concentrated by the prostate. Evidence exists that alcohol contained within the prostate can build to a concentration as much as ten times greater than in the bloodstream. Heavy drinkers often suffer from serious prostate irritation and acute prostate attacks, especially after binges. However, there is no proven link between alcohol and prostate tumors. As mentioned, alcohol is also a factor in impotence and its diuretic effect does add to incontinence problems.

Alcohol should always be used in moderation, but an occasional glass of beer or wine should not be a problem for most nonalcoholic men. Incidentally, red wine appears to be somewhat more irritating to the prostate than white.

Caffeine—present in coffee, tea, cocoa, many soft drinks, and chocolate candy—is a central nervous system stimulant. Tolerance to caffeine varies among individuals, but in some persons even relatively moderate quantities can cause insomnia, nervousness, anxiety, headache, heart palpitations, and diarrhea. Concern has been raised about caffeine in connection with heart attacks, high blood pressure, and stomach ulcers.

Caffeine travels easily to the prostate, where it can cause irritation. As a diuretic, caffeine will also aggravate incontinence. The drug is at its highest concentrations in brewed, nondecaffeinated coffee. I recommend you limit your brewed coffee consumption to no more than two cups a day and restrict your consumption of other caffeine-containing products to moderate levels.

Drugs That Can Irritate the Prostate

Many drugs sold by prescription or over the counter will cause prostate irritation. Whole classes of drugs have been implicated, including antihistamines, anabolic steroids, heart and high blood pressure medications, medications for treating gastrointestinal problems, tranquilizers, and antidepressants. Many of these drugs have also been linked to impotence. Of course, not all drugs in these categories will cause prostate irritation or impotence.

Antihistamines cause some of the most frequent problems, because they are readily available in nonprescription preparations for treating the common cold and allergies. Antihistamines trigger contractions of smooth muscles in the vicinity of the prostate and the bladder. These drugs can also be a factor in impotence and incontinence. In general, they should always be used with proper precautions.

In accordance with good medical practice, any physician should carefully review with you the possible side effects of every drug prescribed for any medical condition. If you have a history of prostate irritation, always ask specifically about any possible side effects relating to the prostate, because that could easily be overlooked by physicians who are not urologists. You can also consult the *Physicians' Desk Reference* (PDR), an annual reference on pharmaceutical products published by the Medical Economics Company, Oradell, New Jersey. The volume is available in most public libraries.

If you develop prostate irritation or any other noticeable side effect while taking a prescribed drug, call your physician at once. An effective alternative drug should be available with fewer side effects. But unless the side effects are really severe, always consult with your physician before you discontinue a prescribed drug.

Given the inherent difficulty of research, information on the possible involvement of the most common illegal drugs in prostate disorders is limited. As mentioned in Chapter 7, there is a known connection between amphetamine or cocaine use and impotence. Therefore, it is not unreasonable to suspect these substances could also adversely impact the prostate. Amphetamines and cocaine are nervous system stimulants with effects that sometimes resemble caffeine, but are usually more severe. This suggests that amphetamines and cocaine, as with caffeine, can irritate the prostate.

Marijuana (cannabis) is the most widely used illegal substance. The drug is known to lower testosterone levels, which, in turn, can cause erection problems. But that might suggest a positive medical role for the drug in treating prostate tumors. There is no evidence that marijuana causes prostate irritation. Morphine, an opium derivative, is widely used in hospitals to relieve postoperative pain. There is no evidence that morphine causes prostate irritation in the hospital setting.

Alternative Medicine

Alternative medicine may be defined as any form of medical treatment that has not met with general approval by the "medical establishment," the network of licensed physicians and surgeons, scientifically trained investigators at recognized medical research institutions, and government regulatory bodies, such as the Food and Drug Administration (FDA).

An important characteristic of alternative medicine is frequent, recommended use of herbs and various plant extracts. Often, the individuals recommending these products also sell them. Under law, such products are usually classed as foods and, unless there are serious health safety factors, their sale is not generally prevented by law, although making specific medical claims for them is usually prohibited by FDA regulations.

When unconventional therapy was broadly construed to include such things as exercise and faith healing, a 1993 survey of 1,500 medical consumers published in the *New England Journal of Medicine* estimated that one in three people used an unconventional therapy, but most frequently as adjuncts to conventional therapy. Most did not tell their physician they were using an unconventional therapy.

My patients frequently hear about alternative treatments for their prostate problems, most of which involve herbs or drugs that have not been approved by the medical establishment. Recently, Ernie, who was being treated for benign prostate enlargement, brought to my attention a thin booklet authored by a Salem Kirban with the title, *The Medical Approach versus The Nutritional Approach to Prostate*

Problems. The booklet contained a section attributed to a Dr. Paul Eck, described as having a degree in "naprapathy," and the director of a laboratory in Arizona specializing in the interpretation of hair tests. Naprapathy is defined in the booklet as "a system of therapy which attributes all disease to disorders of the nervous system, ligaments, and connective tissue," something that would come as quite a surprise to Louis Pasteur, Joseph Lister, and the other great medical pioneers who demonstrated the role of microorganisms in many types of illness. In his section, Dr. Eck states that prostate problems are attributable to "one or more mineral ratio imbalances" that can presumably be identified by hair analysis and corrected by changing those imbalances. In other sections of the book, it is suggested that prostate disorders can be helped by injecting into the rectum, at least three times a day, a half glass of freshly squeezed wheat grass juice or by soaking the buttocks in a cold water bath containing ice cubes. Anxious to help himself, Ernie was quite legitimately worried he was missing out on something useful. He wasn't.

In counseling Ernie, I pointed out, as previously discussed in this chapter, that while zinc and possibly magnesium would appear to be an important factor in prostate metabolism, there is no credible scientific evidence that would support the hope that his BPH condition could be miraculously cured by tampering with the mineral ratio in his body. I also advised that very little is known as to how mineral ratio values, derived from hair sample tests, correlate with the actual balance of minerals within the prostate and, therefore, are in all likelihood useless. As to wheat grass injections, my advice to Ernie was that, other than perhaps causing irritation in the rectal area, it wouldn't hurt. It also wouldn't help. I strongly urged Ernie to forget about ice cube sitz baths. As indicated in Chapter 4, this would be a good way to trigger an episode of very unpleasant prostate irritation.

How then should we view alternative medicine?

Always Keep an Open Mind, but Be Cautious

Whenever you evaluate alternative medicine suggestions, always keep an open mind. The medical establishment has often been highly resistant to change, even to suggestions put forward by its own members. Dr. Ignaz Philipp Semmelweis, a nineteenth-century Hungarian physician, was vilified by his colleagues and hounded from his post at a Vienna maternity hospital when he suggested that the death of many mothers from "childbed" (puerperal) fever was being caused by the failure of physicians to wash their hands between patient examinations. Today, Semmelweis is considered one of the great physicians in the history of medicine.

Many important drugs used by mainstream medicine today were derived originally from herbal sources. Awareness of their value often meant centuries of trial-and-error experimentation by folk healers. Because plants are remarkable chemical factories and can synthesize some very complex substances, it is reasonable that a significant percentage of such substances has been found to have useful medicinal properties.

While I've stressed the importance of an open mind as to alternative medicine claims, it is no contradiction to emphasize that these claims should be assessed cautiously and subjected to scientific evaluation. That implies carefully controlled experiments, full disclosure in appropriate scientific publications of experimental procedures and results, the ability of independent investigators to reproduce experimental results, and critical peer reviews.

Exercise special caution in evaluating alternative prostate treatments, in view of the lengthy history of quackery in the field, most likely a reflection of the link between the prostate and sexuality. Around 1900, a British firm made a fortune selling a foul nostrum called "Swamp Root," said, among other things, to cure prostate enlargement. An analysis showed the product was mostly caramel-colored sugar water. The FDA only recently issued a ban on over-the-counter products that make unsubstantiated claims for treating prostate enlargement.

Suggested Alternative Prostate Remedies

Alternative remedies for treating prostate problems that you hear about most frequently are discussed below. Before you try any of them, speak to your urologist. They could be dangerous if you fail to begin or if you abandon the medically recognized treatment program recommended. Be absolutely sure an alternative remedy has no toxic or allergic side effects that will interfere in any way with the treatment suggested by your urologist. Other factors: Is the remedy legally available and what is its cost?

A useful source on many herbal drugs is *The Merck Index,* published by Merck & Co., Inc., and available in most public or university libraries. Data is provided on chemical properties, sources, therapeutic uses, and toxicity and other possible dangers.

Bee Pollen

When honey bees enter flowers in search of nectar, pollen collects on their bodies. Bee pollen producers recover this pollen by placing wire brushes around the entrance to bee hives. When bees return, they touch the brushes and the pollen falls off. This pollen is collected and pressed into tablets.

Interest in bee pollen was stimulated greatly when it was revealed during the course of the 1972 Munich Olympics that Finnish double gold-medal winner, Lasse Viren (5k and 10k), used the tablets to improve his performance. Interest was stimulated further by a duplicate performance by Viren at the 1976 games in Montreal.

A bee pollen tablet contains thousands of tiny, single-plant spore grains, and an inert binder. The product provides a mixture of amino acids, vitamins, minerals, and enzymes. The composition varies according to the flowers visited by the bees. Suppliers have claimed bee pollen will improve the speed and endurance of runners, swimmers, and other athletes. Among many other health benefits, suppliers claim bee pollen is an aid in shrinking an enlarged prostate.

Bee pollen is expensive. All its constituents are available in a normal diet and, to date, the claims for it have lacked scientific support. WARNING: Bee pollen can cause life-threatening allergic reactions in susceptible individuals.

Buchu

Buchu is an herbal product made by drying the leaves of two closely related plants that grow at the Cape of Good Hope (the southern tip of South Africa). The most important constituent of the leaves is diophenol, also known as barosma camphor.

The herb is taken either as tea or in tincture form. Buchu has recognized medical value and has been used as a urinary antiseptic and diuretic. Claims have been made that Buchu is of some value in treating prostate enlargement, dropsy, rheumatism, and early diabetes. There are no reported toxic effects.

Ginseng

Ginseng is an ancient Chinese remedy obtained from the root of the *Panax ginseng* plant native to China and Korea. However, the United States is now a major producer, with most exported to the Far East. The most important constituent is a resinous material, panaxatriol, which has a steroid nucleus. Ginseng is usually sold in tablets that can be crushed and made into a fairly tasty tea.

There is an important connection between ginseng and the ancient Chinese philosophical concept of yin and yang, according to which the universe consists of two opposing elements. Yin, the female element, stands for cold, darkness, and death. Yang, the male element, stands for warmth, light, and life. Disease is believed to be caused by an imbalance of yin and yang in your body. Taking ginseng is said to restore the balance.

Claims are made that ginseng will help relieve the symptoms of prostate enlargement and urinary-tract inflammation, restore potency, and cure almost everything else that ails you. There is very little clinical proof of such claims, but it is reasonable to ask why the Chinese have persisted in using ginseng for 3,000 years. One explanation is that the connection between ginseng and Chinese religious philosophy makes ginseng, in effect, a form of faith healing. Belief in its effectiveness is sustained by the observation that faith healing, on occasion, does effect cures, especially in individuals whose problems are largely psychosomatic.

The steroids in ginseng can be harmful to some persons. Some problems have been reported, including diarrhea, mental confusion, insomnia, nervousness, skin rashes, and breast enlargement.

Juniper Berry

The herb juniper berry is obtained from the dried ripe fruit, wood, and tops of the juniper plant, *Juniperus communis*. The principal constituent is a volatile oil.

Juniper berry is a diuretic, said to help relieve prostate disorders, skin rashes, and hemorrhoids. The product is also said to kill intestinal worms and is used commercially in fumigants used as pesticides.

Juniper berries are edible and are also used to produce a liqueur. High levels can cause urinary irritation.

Laetrile

Laetrile is the trade name for a drug obtained by processing amygdalin, a complex chemical containing cyanide processed from bitter almonds and the seeds of apricots and peaches. Laetrile has also been referred to as vitamin B_{17}.

Amygdalin's use in cancer chemotherapy has been reported in the medical literature since 1845, the theory being that the cyanide in the substance will kill cancer cells. Recently, Laetrile has created considerable controversy with proponents of the product, claiming successful results, including its use in treating prostate cancer. By applying considerable political pressure, these efforts have had considerable success at the state level. However, the FDA has managed to impose restrictions severely limiting availabilty of Laetrile and these restrictions have been upheld by the U.S. Supreme Court. Some people, however, have attempted to get around FDA restrictions by seeking treatment in Mexico or by eating large quantities of peach and apricot pits and almonds.

Repeated scientific studies have failed to demonstrate that Laetrile has any value at all in treating any form of cancer. Public authorities fear that many persons will choose ineffective Laetrile treatment over conventional treatment that may yield positive results. It should be noted that there have been reports of serious cyanide poisoning and even death in individuals who have eaten large quantities of peach and apricot pits and almonds.

Pumpkin Seed

Pumpkin seed is obtained by drying the ripe seeds of cultivated varieties of the pumpkin plant, especially *Cucurbita pepo* and *Cucurbitaceae*. The most important constituent is oil of pumpkin, a fixed (nonvolatile) oil.

Pumpkin seed has a recognized medical use as an antihelminthic, an agent for eliminating intestinal worms. There have been unsubstantiated claims that worm colonies in the lower bowel can cause prostate enlargement. It is not unreasonable to believe that an infestation of worms in the lower part of the body would add to the general discomfort of men with prostate enlargement. Pumpkin seed can be tasty and no toxic effects are reported from eating moderate quantities.

Raw Vegetable Juices

Claims are frequently made for the health benefits of regularly drinking fresh-squeezed vegetable and fruit juices. One such claim is that regularly drinking a combination of fresh-squeezed cucumber, beet, carrot, and parsley juice will aid the prostate, the kidneys, and other organs.

In the above combination, cucumber juice is known to be diuretic and that may be a problem in individuals with incontinence. Other than that, there shouldn't be any undesirable effects if you take the mixture, and the juices do provide various necessary vitamins and minerals, including beta carotene.

Saw Palmetto

Saw palmetto is an herb obtained from the dwarf palmetto fan palm tree. There have been claims that the herb and its extracts tones and strengthens glandular and muscular tissue, thus helping to treat disorders of the urinary-genital system, including prostate enlargement.

Clinical verification has not been established and the herb is fairly expensive. There are no reported toxic effects.

Permixon is an over-the-counter drug which contains fatty acids extracted from saw palmetto. Other herbal remedies that are sometimes recommended for the prostate include pygeum or pygeum africanum which is used like saw palmetto, as a treatment for prostate enlargement. Ashwaganda or withania somnifera is sometimes recommended as a treatment for sexual deficiency. Ashwaganda is an Ayurvedic or Indian folk medicine remedy, and the plant contains natural steroids, which one study showed to have an anti-inflammatory action and to suppress granulation in the prostates of animals.

Shark Cartilage

A best-selling book has been written on the far-fetched idea that since sharks don't get cancer, people might benefit from taking shark cartilage tablets, which are selling briskly at health food stores. Cartilage is an early and different form of bone; the skeletons of sharks are made from cartilage since they developed relatively early as a life form on earth. Cartilage does contain a protein that blocks the formation of blood vessels, and one test on rabbits showed that some induced tumors in rabbit ears stopped growing when pellets containing cartilage were implanted in their ears. No scientific proof exists that ingesting this substance actually helps prevent or cure any type of cancer, although tests are underway to test this substance on prostate cancer and Kaposi's sarcoma. So far, there have been no reports that this substance is harmful to the human body.

"Vitamin" F

"Vitamin" F dates back to 1932, when two researchers published a paper claiming linoleic and linolenic acids, both unsaturated fatty acid substances found in linseed and other vegetable oils, were essential in human nutrition and, among other benefits, would help prevent kidney damage. In 1934, a paper appeared in which the two acids were designated vitamin F.

Attempts to verify the essential role of linoleic and linolenic acids have failed and the name vitamin F has been discredited. Nevertheless, there have been periods of commercial interest in linoleic and linolenic acids, the earliest during the thirties. More recently, claims have been made that taking the product will help prevent or relieve various forms of cancer, including prostate.

Claims that linoleic and linolenic acid have anticancer properties have yet to be clinically proven. There have been reports that linolenic acid is converted to eicosapentaenoic acid, a product found in fish oils. Evidence exists that fish oils can be a factor in preventing heart disease, but no link has been made with cancer. No serious side effects from ingesting linoleic and linolenic acids are reported.

Prostate Problem Support Groups

You, your partner if you have one, and concerned close family members may benefit by participating in a support group dedicated to some type of prostate problem. Support groups are self-help organizations made up of everyday people affected by the mutual problem. Assistance is provided to support groups on a continuing basis through participation by professional advisers, including physicians, nurses, and social workers. Typically, support groups meet regularly at facilities provided by hospitals, schools, and community centers.

Support groups for wives of prostate cancer patients also exist in some hospitals, and many groups encourage family participation. In communities where support groups do not exist, groups are sometimes started by a urologist who takes an interest, sends out a mailing to patients with prostate cancer, and invites them to attend a meeting. Medical speakers such as nurses or radiation therapists may be asked to address the group. If enough men take an interest, they typically take over the operations of the support group and the urologist falls back into an advisory role. Support groups are not for everybody, but they can help many people cope with the psychological burdens of illness and provide companionship and much-needed support.

A recent Gallup survey of prostate cancer patients found that almost 60 percent of men surveyed had at least tried to participate in a support group. This indicates that it is not unusual for men to seek support at this point in their lives.

Many men surveyed participated in support groups in their local communities, or at hospitals or clinics. The most common membership was in US-TOO, named by more than one-third of the men. When asked how support groups had helped them, 49 percent of respondents said the group provided information, and 51 percent said it brought them together with other people who had experienced prostate cancer. In addition, 13 percent of the men responded that support groups helped them understand their condition better. About 10 percent said the group helped relieve their concerns or fears, and 9 percent said the support group gave them useful information about their treatment options.

As evidence that support groups really do educate people who participate in them, the survey also found that more patients involved in support groups understood the most recent possible treatment options such as cryosurgery or hormone therapy which could be employed for treating aspects of their disease.

Two support groups for coping with prostate cancer now have chapters or representatives in most major American urban centers and, in some cases, outside the United States: Patient Advocates for Advanced Cancer Treatments (PAACT) and US-TOO. A national group known as Impotents Anonymous (IA) provides support for men with impotence problems. Help for Incontinent People (HIP) supports individuals with incontinence. In the appendix of this book, names, addresses, and telephone numbers are listed so that you can contact the nearest group relevant to your condition. Some support groups are conducted by local hospitals or medical groups. Your local newspaper may contain notices or advertisements announcing the time and place of these meetings.

Support group participants come from all walks of life. A typical monthly or bi-monthly meeting begins with an educational talk by the group's medical adviser. Following that, there may be a presentation by an invited professional guest or an educational videocassette. The issues usually discussed by medical experts include treatment options, relevant financial concerns, and coping with emotional difficulties. The rest of each meeting, and perhaps their most important segment, consists typically of open discussion among the participants.

Most support group members find them very helpful. The groups can provide valuable practical information, including where innovative treatments are available, how to participate in field trials of new treatments, and where to get financial assistance. Their emotional support can be equally important. Participants often find they are not alone with their problems and that knowledge can prove most comforting.

In the appendices you'll find more useful self-help information.

There are still no fully effective techniques for preventing most prostate problems, especially benign prostate enlargement and prostate cancer, so early detection and prompt treatment are your best defense, as emphasized repeatedly in this book.

I hope sincerely that you find this book helpful in dealing with a part of your body inherently prone to medical difficulties. I'd be delighted to hear your questions, comments, and suggestions about this book. Stay well.

Your Healthy Prostate Diet

Planning Your Diet

This section contains suggested menus, covering a one-week period, based on a diet that will be kind to your prostate. In it, I recommend foods you should eat regularly, on a limited or occasional basis, and those you should avoid. There are also some tips on eating out and other special problems.

From what we know scientifically about the effect of dietary substances on the prostate and about nutritional principles generally, a diet good for your prostate and for your overall health should:

- Provide an optimum balance of protein, carbohydrates, and fats
- Have low cholesterol levels and relatively high levels of polyunsaturated fat
- Include adequate fiber
- Contain an adequate supply of vitamins, especially vitamin A (preferably as beta carotene), vitamin C, and vitamin E
- Offer an adequate supply of minerals, especially zinc, the prostate mineral
- Limit certain foods and beverages that irritate the prostate
- Always be varied, interesting, and tasty

The menu suggestions provide for a daily caloric intake in the 2,000 to 2,500 calorie range. That level is suitable for a reasonably active man of average height and build. If you are very active or you work outdoors in very cold weather, you may need a daily diet of 3,000 calories or even more. By contrast, if you are overweight, your physician may advise you to cut your intake to 1,800 or even to 1,200 calories until a proper weight is attained. Remember, obesity is bad for your prostate. You can adjust your own calorie intake to the desired level by increasing or reducing the portions in the menus.

One Week of Tasty Eating That Is Good for Your Prostate

MONDAY

Breakfast
Orange juice – large glass
Oatmeal with skim milk – one bowl
Rye bread with jelly – two slices
Coffee or tea – one cup only

Lunch
Split pea soup – one bowl
Mixed tossed salad with olive oil and vinegar – one cup
English muffin with jelly – one
Apple – one
Tomato juice – one small glass

Snack
Banana – one
Pretzel – one

Dinner
Apricot juice and soda – one large glass
Chicken (skinned) baked with banana, onion slices, and fine herbs – 5-oz. portion
Mixed broccoli and cauliflower with grated parmesan cheese – one cup
Boiled potatoes with parsley – two small
Pumpernickel bread – one slice
Fresh peach – one

TUESDAY

Breakfast
Fresh papaya – one medium slice
Fresh pineapple – two slices
Fresh orange – one
Banana – one
Hard roll with mozzarella cheese (low-fat) – one
Coffee or tea – one cup only

Lunch
Minestrone soup – one cup
Turkey on rye sandwich with cold slaw and Russian dressing – one
Kosher-style pickle – one
Skim milk – one cup

Snack
Celery – three pieces
Raisins – ¼ cup

Dinner

Clam juice – one glass

Shrimp Creole – Eight shrimp with sauce of onions, bell peppers, tomatoes, and mushrooms sautéed with olive oil

Steamed rice – one cup

Carrot salad – one cup

Garlic bread – two slices

Fresh stawberries – ½ cup

WEDNESDAY

Breakfast

Vegetable juice – one large glass

Poached egg on rye toast – one

Extra slice of rye bread with jelly

Grits – ½ cup

Coffee or tea – one cup only

Lunch

Chilled half grapefruit – one

Black beans, chopped onions, and pimentoes over rice – one bowl

Hard roll – one

Skimmed milk – one cup

Snack

Graham crackers – two

Grapes – medium bunch

Dinner

Mixed fruit juices and soda – one glass

Fresh poached salmon – 6-oz. portion

Small tartar sauce

Watercress salad – one cup

Baked potato with olive oil – one medium

Hard roll – one with margarine

Stewed rhubarb – ½ cup

THURSDAY

Breakfast

Orange juice – one large glass

Raisin bran cereal with banana – one bowl

Pumpernickel bread with jelly – one slice

Coffee or tea – one cup only

Lunch

Onion soup with parmesan cheese – one bowl

Pickled herring salad – four ounces on bed of lettuce

Hard roll with margarine – one

Mixed fruit juice – one large glass

Snack

Popcorn – one cup

Dinner

Cranberry juice – one large glass

Chicken (5 oz., skinned) stir fried with Chinese vegetables

Thai-style rice noodles – one cup

Mixed fresh fruit – one cup

FRIDAY

Breakfast

Orange juice – one large glass
Yogurt (low-fat) – one cup
Rye bread with jelly – two slices
Coffee or tea – one cup only

Lunch

Seafood gumbo – one cup
Grilled tomato and bleu cheese on sliced English muffin
Mixed tossed salad with olive oil and vinegar – one cup
Skim milk – one cup

Snack

Pear – one
Rice crackers – two

Dinner

White wine – one glass (recognizing "TGIF")
Sirloin steak (extra lean) with mushroom caps – 4-oz. portion
Brussels sprouts – ½ cup
Lettuce salad
French bread – one slice
Mixed fresh fruit – one cup

SATURDAY

Breakfast

Vegetable juice – one small glass
Omelet with one egg, tofu, and mixed vegetables – one cup
Pumpernickel bread with jelly – two slices
Coffee or tea – one glass

Lunch

Wonton soup – one bowl
Tomato stuffed with tuna fish salad (3 oz. tuna fish, chopped onions, celery, parsley, and two tablespoons of mayonnaise)

Hard roll – one
Banana
Iced tea – one glass

Dinner

Mixed alcoholic drink – one glass (it's Saturday night)
Broiled swordfish – 4-oz. portion
Cooked spinach – one cup
Rice – ½ cup
Sherbet – ½ cup

SUNDAY

Breakfast

Smoked salmon – ¼ ounce
Cream cheese – two tablespoons
Bagels – two
Coffee or tea – one cup only

Lunch

Lentil soup – one cup
Pasta salad – one cup
Rye bread – one slice

Apple – one
Skimmed milk – one glass

Dinner

Fruit juice with soda – one large glass
Baked turkey wing with celery, onions, and parsley – 5 oz.
Braised carrots – two
Mashed potatoes – ½ cup
Angel food cake – one slice

Good Foods to Eat

The above menus provide a healthy pattern for your weekly diet. You can stick to that pattern, but at the same time, add variety to your diet by making substitutions in each food area based on the following list:

High-Fat Foods

- Margarine made only from corn, sunflower, or liquid safflower oils
- Cooking or salad oils high in monounsaturated fats—olive and peanut oil. *Caution:* don't use peanut oil if you have a peanut allergy
- Cooking or salad oils high in polyunsaturated fats—corn, soybean, sunflower, and safflower oils

High-Protein Foods

- Red meats—use only lean and well-trimmed beef, veal, pork, and lamb (limit, 7 oz. a day). *Note:* most game is low fat
- Fish
- Shellfish—Moderate servings only
- Skinless chicken and turkey
- Tofu, dried beans, peas, and peanut butter (unless allergic)

Dairy Products

- Liquid milk—use only skimmed or 1 percent low-fat
- Dried milk—low- or nonfat only
- Low-fat cheeses—cottage, mozzarella, ricotta, and other white cheeses
- Ice milk, sherbet, and sorbet
- Low-fat yogurt

High-Carbohydrate Foods

- Rye, pumpernickel, and whole wheat breads
- English muffins, bagels, and plain rolls
- Hot and cold breakfast cereals

- Low-fat baked goods—graham and soda crackers, angel food cake, pretzels, and rice cakes
- Popcorn (no added oil or butter)

Fruits and Vegetables

- Raw fruits and vegetables
- Vegetables boiled, baked, steamed, or microwaved with only small amounts of suitable oils
- Lightly stir-fried vegetables

Some Foods to Limit

It is best to consume the following foods only on special occasions or in limited quantities:

High-Fat Foods

- Butter
- Margarine manufactured from hydrogenated oils
- Vegetable shortenings made from hydrogenated or partially hydrogenated vegetable oils
- Shortening made from lard and other meat fats
- Chocolate
- Cheese and sour cream salad dressings

High-Protein Foods

- Fatty meats—high-fat hamburger, marbled beef, sausage, bacon, and most processed cold cuts
- Fried chicken and fish

- Unskinned chicken
- Goose and duck
- Liver

Dairy Products

- High-fat milk
- Light and whipped cream
- High-fat ice cream
- Whole sour cream and yogurt
- High-fat cheeses

High-Carbohydrate Foods

- Most snack foods—potato chips, cheese crackers, and pork rinds
- Most doughnuts, pastries, pies, cakes, and cookies
- Pasta and rice products high in fats

Fruits and Vegetables

- Avocado
- Vegetables cooked in butter, lard, hydrogenated shortenings, and deep fat
- Vegetables seasoned with butter, cream sauces, and chunks of pork fat

Foods and Beverages
Known to Irritate the Prostate

- Coffee, tea, and soft drinks containing caffeine
- Alcohol
- Very spicy foods

Some Foods to Avoid

It is best to avoid or severely limit your consumption of these foods:

- Coconuts; coconut cakes, cookies, and candies; and coconut oil
- Margarines and shortenings made from coconut, palm, and palm kernel oils
- Lard and beef tallow
- Cocoa butter
- Heavy cream

Eating Out and Other Problems

There is no greater threat to your healthy prostate than a typical American restaurant's food. Although there should be no real problem when eating out in getting all the zinc and other important minerals and vitamins you need in your diet, chances are that unless you choose to go hungry, it will take your best efforts to avoid excess cholesterol and saturated fats.

If you have a good diet at home and only eat out on special occasions, enjoy yourself and don't worry. Occasionally, going off your diet within reason should usually have no measurable effect on your prostate and will even serve as a reward for your good behavior the rest of the time. You will have a problem if your work requires you to travel extensively or you have frequent business meals. Here are some tips for dealing with this problem:

- Breakfast is the most challenging meal. A typical restaurant breakfast menu limits your choice to eggs, bacon and sausage, and pancakes containing eggs. Check to see if there are any cereals or fresh fruit. If not, ask for English muffins with margarine or go up the street and buy something good to eat in your room.
- Look for ethnic restaurants, especially those serving Asian, Italian, and Mexican food. Asian cuisine, including Chinese, Japanese, Thai, and Indian, is typically a

mixture of vegetables over a bed of rice or noodles. Meat is used mainly as a seasoning. You should be careful, however, with highly spiced Thai food, and some regional Chinese and Indian foods cooked with coconut oil. Italian food is typically low in fat and ideally cooked with olive oil. Mexican food, other than guacamole (contains avocado) and items with sour cream, is usually good for you and tasty.

- Look for seafood or vegetarian restaurants. In a seafood restaurant, limit your entrée to baked or broiled items and avoid breaded and deep fried foods. Vegetarian and health food restaurants sometimes serve interesting food, but be careful of items containing cheese and sour cream.

- Unless you are in a fast food restaurant where there is little choice about how food is prepared, ask how they do it, and, if necessary, ask to have your meal prepared in a healthier manner.

- Avoid salad bars and buffets, because you'll tend to eat too much, and many of the prepared items are loaded with cholesterol. And remember: that familiar plastic panel you see at salad bars is a "sneeze shield." But the heads of most children and some short adults are often below it.

- If you are flying, check with your airline in advance to see if they serve special meals, especially seafood, vegetable, and fresh fruit entrées. If not, eat selectively from the food you are served.

Finally, there are the endless problems with annual holidays such as Thanksgiving and Christmas, special family occasions, office parties, and social events. There is no easy solution. My best advice is to accept the inevitable, but afterward promptly resume your healthy diet. Continuing to maintain your exercise program, as discussed in other chapters, will also help.

A Basic Prostate Glossary

A

Acid phosphatase: Enzyme produced only in the prostate. High levels may indicate the spread of prostate cancer. See prostatic acid phosphatase (PAP) test.

Acute prostatitis: Prostate infection characterized by the sudden flare-up of severe symptoms such as high fever and a burning feeling when urinating, which usually run their course in a relatively short time.

Adenocarcinoma: Malignant (cancerous) tumor with a foothold within a gland or body part with a glandular structure.

Adenoma: Benign tumor within a gland or body part with a glandular structure.

Adenomectomy: Surgical removal of excess tissue from a gland harboring a benign tumor.

Adrenal glands: Two small ductless glands located near the kidneys. Adrenal glands secrete epinephrine, cortisone, and the androgen hormone testosterone.

Alpha adrenergic blocker: Class of drugs used to treat benign prostate enlargement that tend to relax the smooth muscles of the prostate and, if effective, improve urine flow. These drugs are also used to treat hypertension. The best known alpha adrenergic blocker is sold under the name Hytrin. This drug is awaiting FDA approval for BPH treatment.

Androgen hormone: Hormonal substance produced in the body that is essential for proper development and functioning of the male sexual organs and secondary male sexual characteristics such as deep voice, facial hair, and muscular build. Testosterone is the most important androgen hormone.

Antiandrogen drug: Any drug that reduces or totally blocks the normal activity of an androgen hormone. Antiandrogen drugs have a role in treating both benign and malignant prostate tumors.

Antibacterial drug: Drug used to treat an infection caused by some form of bacteria. Most common prostate infections are caused by bacteria and are treated with antibacterial drugs.

Antibiotic: Drug usually produced from living organisms that helps cure infections caused by bacteria. A broad-spectrum antibiotic is effective against many types of bacteria. A narrow-spectrum antibiotic is effective against a limited number of bacterial types.

Antifungal: A drug used against fungus organisms that cause vaginal yeast infections in women that can also cause corresponding infections of the male prostate.

Antihistamine: Drug used mainly to treat various allergies caused by the presence in the body of histamine, a substance that builds up in the body from an allergic reaction. Antihistamines usually cause some increased difficulty in urination.

Anti-inflammatory: Drug that helps reduce pain, swelling, heat, and other irritation resulting from infection or other causes such as prostatosis or prostatodynia.

Anus: Muscular opening to the body at the downstream end of the rectum; outlet for solid body waste.

Artificial sphincter: Prosthesis or artificial device sometimes used to treat incontinence after prostate surgery. An artificial sphincter substitutes for natural urinary sphincter muscles that normally control the urine flow from the bladder.

B

Bacteria: Microscopic one-celled plants. Some bacteria are harmless or even beneficial; others can cause infection. Most prostate infections are caused by common forms of bacteria found in the gastrointestinal system.

Balloon dilatation: Nonsurgical procedure, also known as balloon urethroplasty, used to treat benign prostate enlargement. An inflatable balloon is inserted in that region of the urethra constricted by excess prostatic tissue. Its inflation improves urine flow.

Behavior therapy: Treatment system in which patients are subjected systematically to psychological conditioning in the hope that this will eliminate pain and discomfort that may not be the result of an actual physical problem such as prostatodynia.

Benign: Term describing a medical condition generally favorable for recovery, not always permanently damaging, and noncancerous (nonmalignant).

Benign prostate hypertropy (BPH): Older and no-longer-preferred name for condition known as benign prostatic hyperplasia.

Benign prostatic hyperplasia (BPH): Condition characterized by growth of a benign tumor inside the prostate, often resulting in voiding difficulties. Also known as benign prostate hypertrophy.

Benign tumor: Noncancerous tissue growth that cannot spread from its location site to other areas of the body.

Beta carotene: A form of vitamin A found naturally in many fruits and vegetables; the yellow coloring agent added to margarine. There is increasing evidence that beta carotene has anticancer properties.

Biofeedback: Treatment method based on psychological principles in which patients are trained to control some form of bodily activity by observing sight or sound signals. Biofeedback has been used to treat prostatodynia.

Biopsy: Diagnostic procedure in which a tissue sample is surgically removed from some portion of the body and subjected to microscopic analysis. Most biopsies are performed to determine whether an observed growth of tissue, such as a tumor of the prostate, is malignant or benign.

Bladder: Saclike, stretchable organ, located inside the pelvic cavity for temporary storage of urine produced by the kidneys.

Blood count: Test determining the level of red and white blood cells and platelets in a patient's bloodstream. An abnormal blood count may indicate infection, anemia, or the spread of prostate cancer.

Blood poisoning: Infection caused by invasion of the bloodstream by bacteria or fungi. A treatable complication that sometimes follows prostate surgery. Also, septicemia.

Blood tests: Series of tests on samples of patient's blood that may include a blood count; measurement of sedimentation rate; determination of sugar, cholesterol, and triglyceride levels; diagnosis of presence of infectious organisms; and sometimes special tests of the prostate, such as PSA and PAP assays. Blood tests are sometimes called blood chemistry analysis.

Bone scan: Diagnostic test consisting of a series of X rays of patient's skeletal system. A radioactive substance is injected into the patient during the test to enhance X-ray images. Bone scans can determine whether malignancy has spread from the prostate in patients diagnosed with prostate cancer.

Bulbous urethra: Enlarged section of the urethra downstream from where the urethra passes through the prostate. Seminal fluid collects in the bulbous urethra before ejaculation.

C

Calculus: Hardened, stonelike mass of high calcium content sometimes formed in the kidney, bladder, and prostate. Its plural is calculi. Prostate stones are generally not serious, but may contribute to chronic prostatitis.

Cancer: Family of diseases characterized by uncontrollable cell growth and the ability of this growth to spread from its initial site to other parts of the body. Cancer presents a threat to life when growth crowds out or otherwise interferes with normal function of critical body organs and life-support systems.

Capsule: Term referring to a layer of cells surrounding an organ such as the prostate. Prostate cancer begins to invade other parts of the body when a growing tumor breaks through the prostate capsule.

Carcinogen: Any chemical substance demonstrated by scientific investigation to trigger a genetic defect that results in some form of cancer.

Carcinoma: Most common form of cancer characterized by the growth of a malignant tumor in surface tissues of an organ or on the skin. Prostate cancer is a form of carcinoma.

Castration: Originally, surgical removal of the testes (see orchiectomy). As now used, the term includes elimination of testicular function by administering certain antiandrogen drugs.

Catheter: Flexible tube inserted into some part of the body that provides a channel for fluid passage or a medical device. Depending on circumstances, a catheter may remove waste fluids from the body after a transurethral resection (TURP).

Chemotherapy: Treatment for cancer based on use of various potent drugs that attack and destroy certain types of cancer. Such drugs are either injected or taken orally and often produce side effects.

Chlamydia: Infectious microorganism associated most often with vaginal infections in women; characterized by a whitish discharge from the penis. Chlamydia can be sexually transmitted and can also cause a form of prostatitis.

Cholesterol: Chemical substance of the steroid type produced naturally in the body or ingested from certain foods. A minimum quantity of cholesterol is needed by the body, but an excess can cause various health problems, including cardiovascular disease and gallstones. Cholesterol in the diet has been linked to both benign prostate enlargement and to prostate cancer.

Chronic prostatitis: Persistent form of prostatitis lasting for an extended period—sometimes years. Chronic prostatitis usually has fairly mild symptoms that may, at times, be acute.

Circumcision: Surgical procedure in men consisting of removing the foreskin (portion of the forward tip) of the penis. A religious practice of Jews, Moslems, and some others. In the United States, most males are routinely circumcized.

Clinical trials: Research studies performed on patients to determine effectiveness of new drugs or other medical treatments. Patients who volunteer for clinical trials must read and sign a statement indicating "informed consent." For research purposes, some patients may receive a placebo in a clinical trial, instead of the drug under investigation.

Coitus interruptus: Form of birth control in which a man withdraws his penis from a women's vagina before ejaculation. As a birth control method, the practice is unreliable and may contribute to prostate congestion and resulting irritation.

Coliform bacteria: Class of bacteria normally found in gastrointestinal systems of humans and other animals. Coliform bacteria can invade the prostate where they cause the most common type of prostate infection.

Collagen: Colloidal chemical substance made of proteins, sometimes injected into the urinary sphincter region to treat incontinence.

Colon: Lower section of the large intestine leading into the rectum. (Coliform bacteria are so named owing to their presence in high numbers in the colon.)

Computerized tomography: Also called CT scan; an X-ray technique employing modern computer technology to enhance image quality. CT is valuable for examining soft body tissue.

Congestion: Situation characterized by buildup of fluid in some area of the body. In prostate congestion, there is an unrelieved, often painful buildup of prostatic fluid in the prostate, sometimes accounting for cases of prostatosis.

Contraindication: Term that identifies a medical situation created when a given drug or some medical treatment is not recommended because of undesirable side effects.

Corpus cavernosagram: Test used in treatment of impotence in which a special dye is injected into a patient's penis so that a series of X rays can be taken of the organ's interior structure. May reveal the location of leaking veins responsible for the inability to sustain an erection.

Corpus cavernosum: Body of tissue inside the penis containing thousands of expandable saclike structures known as sinuses. When the sinuses fill up with blood, an erection results.

Cryosurgery: Surgery that employs extreme cold to destroy undesired tissue. Cryosurgery is being used on a limited basis to treat prostate enlargement and cancer.

Cystoscope: Tubelike device (a type of endoscope) containing a light and viewing lens which, when inserted into the urethra, is used to examine the urethra and bladder in both men and women, and the prostate in men.

Cystoscopy: Diagnostic procedure for urological examination of both men and women. The procedure permits direct viewing by the urologist of the inside of the urinary tract.

D

Diagnosis: Determination by observation or scientific tests of the existence of symptoms that cause a medical disorder.

Digital rectal examination: Highly important prostate examination; the examining physician inserts a gloved finger into a patient's rectum and feels for any abnormality present on the outer lobes of the prostate. The procedure is also used to obtain prostatic fluid samples for laboratory analysis.

Diuretic: Any drug, food, or beverage that promotes increased urine excretion.

DNA probe: Recently developed diagnostic tool based on the application of modern molecular genetics. In the future, DNA probes may provide more accurate, and possibly noninvasive diagnosis of prostate cancer.

Drip collector: Collecting device, either internal or external, to collect urine from an incontinent person.

E

Ejaculate: Fluid that normally passes out of the penis during ejaculation. Ejaculate generally contains sperm originating in the testicles and seminal fluid originating in the testicles, seminal vesicles, and prostate.

Ejaculation: Ejection of sperm and seminal fluid from the penis from contraction of muscles in the urethra and prostate area.

Ejaculatory failure: Failure of a man to ejaculate, despite an extended period of physical and emotional stimulus of the penis.

Electrostimulation: Use of a mild electrical current to stimulate ejaculation or to strengthen muscle action controlling voiding in incontinent persons.

Enzyme: Chemical substance produced naturally in the body that catalyzes or promotes certain essential metabolic processes.

Epididymis: Two common-shaped tubes inside the scrotum that surround each testicle.

Epididymitis: Infection, frequently accompanying cases of prostatitis, of the tubes surrounding the testicles; typically causes pain in the testicles.

Escherichia coli (E. coli): Most common coliform bacteria; the usual cause of prostatitis.

Estrogen: One of the most important sex hormones contributing to development of female sexual characteristics. Large quantities are produced in female ovaries, far lesser amounts in male testicles.

External collection device: Urine collection device used by incontinent individuals to capture urine after it exits the body.

External radiation therapy: Radiation therapy in which X rays or other subatomic particles are focused on cancerous tissue from a source outside the body.

F

5-alpha reductase: Enzyme found in the prostate that controls conversion of testosterone into dihydrotestosterone (DHT). When the action of this enzyme is blocked, production of DHT is inhibited, stopping growth of a benign prostate tumor.

Foley catheter: Type of catheter named for its inventor, with a balloon at the end inserted into the body. The balloon holds the catheter in place. A Foley is usually inserted through the penis to drain urine after prostate surgery.

Foreplay: Erotic physical sexual activity preceding intercourse. Extended foreplay not followed by ejaculation can cause prostate congestion and irritation.

Functional incontinence: Characterized by inability to void in time owing to physical disability or psychological problems. Also, iatrogenic incontinence.

Fungal infection: Infection of prostate or another part of the body caused by a fungus microorganism such as candida.

Fungus: Class of simple plants, including molds, yeast, mushrooms, and mildew. These plants contain no chlorophyll, so they grow parasitically on live hosts or dead organic matter.

G

Gland: Organ of the body that processes chemical substances in the blood to produce other chemical substances for use in the body or for elimination from the body. A gland may have ducts for pouring its secretions into other parts of the body, or it may be ductless and pour secretions into the bloodstream. The prostate is a ducted gland.

Gonorrhea: Sexually transmitted disease characterized by a yellowish discharge from the penis. Also, "the clap." The microorganism that causes gonorrhea may attack the prostate and cause a form of prostatitis.

Groin: Part of the body located along the fold or crease formed where the thighs connect to the lower abdomen.

H

Hematospermia: Frightening but not necessarily serious condition in which blood is found in seminal fluid. Often caused by a prostate infection.

Herb: Plant without woody tissue valued for its medicinal properties or its ability to season food or to provide a pleasant scent.

Herbal medicine: Traditional, prescientific medicine based on herbs. Many effective drugs in the modern pharmacopoeia are the result of the trial and error approach of centuries of herbal medicine.

High blood pressure: Excessive pressure within the bloodstream that results in strain throughout the circulatory system; may cause damage to major organs. Medically, hypertension.

Hormonal therapy: Therapy based on administering certain hormones or chemical substances that block the action of other hormones. In benign prostate enlargement, hormonal therapy blocks the action of male hormones that promote tumor growth.

Hormones: Chemical substances made in various endocrine glands of the body that are essential for certain biological processes.

Hyperthermia: Form of treatment for benign prostate enlargement and prostate cancer that uses high levels of heat produced by microwave radiation to reduce obstruction to urine flow.

I

Imaging studies: Diagnostic studies utilizing photographic images of the prostate produced by X ray or ultrasound. These images may be enhanced by computer or by chemical substances injected into the patient during the test procedure.

Impotence: Inability of a man to achieve or maintain an erection of sufficient duration to satisfy both sexual partners.

Incontinence: Loss of urinary control. Incontinence may be complete or partial and can result from prostate surgery or from radiation therapy for prostate cancer.

Indications: Term that specifies the recommended use or uses of a given drug.

Infertility: In a man with prostate problems, the inability to father a child due to prostate infection or retrograde ejaculation.

Interstitial radiation therapy: Radiation treatment for prostate cancer in which radioactive substances known as "seeds" are implanted within the malignant tumor mass. Also, internal radiation therapy.

Intravenous pyelogram (IVP): Diagnostic technique for examining the urinary system with X-ray images taken after injecting image-enhancing substances into the patient's bloodstream. These injected substances result in greatly improved image quality.

Involution: Term describing changes such as diminished physical vigor or organic functioning in any aging organ such as the prostate.

Irritated prostate: Prostate condition associated with sexual behavior, characterized by pain and other discomfort.

K

Kegel exercises: System of pelvic exercise to diminish or overcome urinary incontinence. Kegel exercise regimens may help eliminate incontinence in men and women, including men with incontinence following prostate surgery.

Kidneys: Two parallel glandular organs located at the back of the abdominal cavity, close to the spinal column. The kidneys separate waste products from blood, excreting them as urine.

L

Lack of desire: Condition, often with a physical cause, characterized by loss of sexual interest or libido.

Laparoscopic lymph node dissection: Test procedure using a device called a laparoscope that involves the removal of tissue through small incisions for later examination of possibly cancerous lymph nodes in the vicinity of the prostate.

Laser: Concentrated and precisely controlled beam of light and energy that can cut away tissue in an operative procedure. The word "laser" is an acronym for "Light Amplification by Stimulated Emission of Radiation."

Lithotropy: Recently developed noninvasive technique that eliminates kidney and urethral calculi (stones) by ultrasound. The technique is not yet suitable for treating prostate stones.

Lower back pain: Pain in the lower region of the back which frequently is due to a prostate disorder. Pain in this area is caused by a prostate problem and is a consequence of the fact that blood veins from the prostate drain into the lower back region.

Luteinizing hormone (LH): Type of hormone produced in the pituitary gland that promotes secretion of male and female sex hormones.

Luteinizing hormone-releasing hormone therapy (LHRH): Prostate cancer treatment in which drugs known as LHRH analogs block testosterone activity, which helps retard tumor growth.

Lymph: Transparent, slightly yellow fluid derived from body tissues throughout the body. Lymph produced in the tissues is conveyed by the lymphatic system into the bloodstream.

Lymphadenectomy: Test procedure performed on patients with diagnosed prostate cancer to determine possible spread of cancerous cells into lymph nodes near the prostate. See "laparoscopic lymph node dissection" and "open pelvic lymph node dissection."

Lymphatic system: Extensive metabolic system consisting of lymph nodes, a network of small vessels called lymphatics that transport lymph, and the large lymph gland known as the spleen. The lymphatic system serves as a vehicle for the spread of prostate cancer. Cancer of the lymphatic system takes two forms, lymphoma and Hodgkin's disease.

Lymph nodes: Small, bean-shaped glands found throughout the trunk of the body and the neck that filter bacteria and toxins from nearby tissues.

M

Magnesium: Metallic mineral essential in the diets of all animals, including humans. Magnesium may play a special role in prostate health.

Magnetic resonance imaging (MRI): Advanced diagnostic technique employing an electromagnetic field and computer analysis that permits examination of soft body tissues including prostate cancers.

Malignancy: Uncontrollable cell growth in some part of the body that can spread to other parts, ultimately causing death. A malignant tumor is cancerous.

Masturbation: Self-stimulation of male or female sexual organs. In the male, masturbation usually results in ejaculation, a process that helps relieve prostate congestion and prevents irritation.

Metastasis: Medical term for the spread through the bloodstream or lymphatic system of a cancer from its original site to other parts of the body. A cancer that has spread is said to have "metastasized."

Mineral: One of about thirty relatively simple chemical substances required in the diets of all animals, including humans. Some minerals are compounds of metals (calcium, iron, sodium, potassium, magnesium, copper, manganese, and zinc). Others are compounds of nonmetals (phosphorous, iodine, sulfur, chlorine, and fluorine).

N

Neoplasm: Any abnormal growth in the body. A neoplasm may be benign or malignant.

Noninfectious prostatitis: Condition characterized by the symptoms of prostatitis, but where no infectious agent can be detected by laboratory analysis. *See* prostatosis and prostatodynia.

O

Obesity: Unhealthy condition defined by the National Institutes of Health as an excess of 20 percent or more of an individual's *body mass index* (BMI), a ratio of an individual's weight and height in kilograms per meter, compared to a normal value in men at age twenty-four.

Open pelvic lymph node dissection: Type of lymphadenectomy requiring a major surgical incision into the body. Most often performed during a radical prostatectomy.

Orchiectomy: Removal by surgery of one or more testicles. *See* castration.

Orgasm: In men, the pleasurable sensations felt in the penis at the moment when muscles in the vicinity of the urethra and pelvic area vigorously contract to force ejaculation of seminal fluid. Men who have had prostate surgery may in some instances fail to ejaculate fluid from the penis, but may still experience the sensation of orgasm. See "retrograde ejaculation."

Outpatient: Treatment that does not involve an overnight hospital stay. May take place in a hospital or a medical office.

Overflow incontinence: Characterized by a temporary inability to void, followed by uncontrollable urine flow. Also, paradoxical incontinence.

P

Pelvic relaxation exercises: Series of exercises involving the pelvic region of the body designed to improve general tone of the prostate and nearby organs.

Pelvic thrusts: Exercise of potential benefit to the prostate involving repeated forward thrusting of the pelvis.

Pelvis: Portion of the skeleton forming a bony girdle joining the lower or hind limbs to the body. The pelvic bones are often a point of attack in men with prostate cancer.

Penile implant: Prosthesis or artificial device used to treat impotence. When surgically inserted into the penis, it provides sufficient rigidity for vaginal penetration and sustained sexual intercourse.

Penile injection therapy: Treatment for impotence involving injection of a drug into the penis resulting in an erection of temporary but sufficient duration for vaginal penetration and intercourse.

Penile warts: Growths on the penis known medically as condylomas, caused by a virus. Penile warts are normally only a minor problem to a man, but have been linked to cervical cancer in their female partners.

Perineal prostatectomy: Prostatectomy in which surgical incision into the body is made through the perineal area, a section of the crotch behind the scrotum and in front of the anus.

Peyronie's disease: Caused by a plaque buildup along the walls of the erectile tissues of the penis. Resulting scarring creates a bend in the penis that may make vaginal penetration impossible or, if achieved, may cause intercourse to be very painful.

Pituitary gland: Gland at the base of the brain that produces hormones stimulating release of other hormones, including testosterone.

Plaque: Buildup of fatty tissue at some point inside the body.

Premature ejaculation: Male sexual dysfunction when ejaculation occurs well before desired by both partners. May be caused by prostatitis.

Priapism: Serious medical emergency characterized by a painful and unwanted erection that persists for an extended period of time.

Primary cancer: Cancer that originates on its own at a specific site in the body, rather than having spread there from another site. Prostate cancer is a primary cancer.

Progression: Term indicating continuing development of a malignancy or its reappearance after apparent disappearance after treatment.

Prolonged ejaculation: Takes place only after an extended period of penis stimulation. May result in prostate congestion.

Prostate: Firm, muscular gland (actually a group of glands) that surrounds the urethra near the outlet of the bladder. The prostate's principal function appears to be manufacturing fluid that constitutes a portion of the semen.

Prostate congestion: *See* "Congestion."

Prostate massage: Stroking and kneading the prostate using a gloved finger inserted through the rectum. Prostate massage is used to obtain a sample of prostatic fluid for laboratory examination or to relieve prostate congestion.

Prostate specific antigen test (PSA): Blood test measuring the level of prostate-specific antigen, a chemical substance produced only in the prostate. A prostate-specific antigen level above normal may indicate prostate enlargement or cancer, and signals prompt further investigation.

Prostate stone: *See* "Calculus."

Prostatectomy: Surgical removal of all or part of the prostate gland.

Prostatic acid phosphatase test (PAP): Blood test performed to determine prostatic acid phosphatase level, a substance produced in the prostate. Elevated PAP levels may indicate the spread of prostate cancer.

Prostatic ducts: Group of twenty to thirty tubes inside the prostate that collect and transport prostatic fluid to the ejaculatory ducts.

Prostatic fluid: Fluid produced by the prostate that accounts for a portion of the semen and is thought to contain chemical substances contributing to the viability of sperm for reproduction.

Prostatitis: Infection of the prostate caused most commonly by coliform bacteria. Prostatitis may be acute or chronic.

Prostatodynia: Condition characterized by pain and other symptoms in the general vicinity of the prostate. As with prostatosis, no infectious microorganism can be detected.

Prostatosis: Disorder of the prostate exhibiting typical symptoms of prostatitis, but where no infectious microorganism can be detected by laboratory analysis.

Pubococcygeus muscles: Group of muscles near the rectum. Kegel exercises are designed to strengthen these muscles and may help to alleviate incontinence in men and women.

R

Radiation therapy: Treatment for cancer involving destruction of malignant tissue growth by bombardment with X rays or other high-energy radiation.

Radical prostatectomy: Form of prostatectomy often used to treat prostate cancer. Involves complete removal of the prostate gland.

Recommended daily allowance (RDA): Based upon the available scientific evidence, quantity of a vitamin or mineral established by the Food and Nutrition Board of the National Academy of Sciences, Washington, D.C., as adequate "to meet the needs of practically all healthy persons." The RDA differs from the Minimum Daily Requirement (MDR), the minimum that must be ingested to prevent dietary deficiency.

Reconstructive surgery: Surgery, the object of which is to restore proper function to some part of the body. May be attempted to treat both impotence and incontinence.

Rectum: Last several inches of the intestines below the colon and above the anus. Repository for solid body waste.

Refractory: Condition referring to a disease that can no longer be controlled by the treatment program in effect. When a prostate cancer is said to be refractory, there is a need for some form of additional treatment.

Resectoscope: Instrument similar to a cystoscope inserted through the tip of the penis to examine an obstruction causing voiding problems and, when indicated, used to perform a transurethral resection of the prostate.

Response: Term indicating an improvement in a patient's condition after some form of treatment. A prostate cancer has a positive "response" when there is a reduction in tumor size or improved blood test readings.

Resting secretion: Usual rate of prostatic fluid secretion in the absence of erotic stimulation. With stimulation and following ejaculation, the prostate increases the production rate to a level higher than the resting-secretion rate.

Retrograde ejaculation: Ejaculation that generally takes place with normal physical sensation, but without the normal flow of semen from the tip of the penis. May occur after prostate surgery.

Retropubic prostatectomy: Prostatectomy is when a surgical incision is made through the abdomen at a point above where the penis enters the body, cutting through the bladder to reach the prostate.

S

Sailor's disease: Irritated prostate condition resulting from prolonged periods of sexual abstinence. Also, "priest's disease."

Schistosomiasis: Serious disease caused by parasitic worms harbored by snails in some Third World countries. The worms can invade the prostate and cause a form of prostatitis.

Scrotum: External pouch of skin containing the testicles and epididymis.

Seeds: Radioactive pellets implanted in the prostate to destroy cancerous growth.

Self-contained penile implant: Penile prosthesis that may be inflated or deflated at will. The entire hydraulic inflation mechanism is contained within the device.

Semen: Cloudy white fluid produced from liquids supplied by the testicles, prostate, and seminal vesicles. The vehicle for carrying sperm.

Seminal vesicles: Two glands located near the prostate that provide a portion of the semen.

Semirigid malleable penile implant: Simplest type of penile prosthesis that can be placed in a straight position before sexual intercourse and otherwise bent downward. A disadvantage: The device results in a semirigid penis.

Sexually transmitted disease: Disease whose principal mode of transmission is sexual activity. An earlier term, "venereal disease," is no longer favored.

Side effect: Undesired symptom that occurs when a patient takes a medication or has some other form of treatment. Impotence may be a side effect of certain drugs used to treat prostate tumors.

Silent BPH: Benign prostatic hyperplasia characterized by growth of a benign tumor in a direction that cannot readily be detected by the digital rectal examination.

Sitz bath: Comforting bath in which the patient sits in a few inches of warm water. Used to treat prostatitis, prostatosis, and prostatodynia.

Sperm: Single, tadpole-shaped cells produced in the testicles and transported by semen. The male genetic contribution to reproduction.

Sphincter: Group of muscles surrounding an opening in the body that expand or contract to control the flow of fluid through the opening. The urinary sphincter at the base of the bladder controls urine flow through the urethra.

Stage: Term describing the size of a malignancy and how far it has spread. There are four stages in prostate cancer, commencing with Stage A, where the malignant tumor is contained entirely within the prostate, ending in Stage D, after the tumor has spread to other parts of the body.

Staging: In prostate cancer, tests that determine the existing stage of the disease and monitor its progress or response.

Staphylococcus: Class of bacteria that causes some cases of prostatitis. Staphylococcus epidemics on occasion occur in hospitals and can complicate patient recovery after prostate surgery.

Steal syndrome: Name given to an impotence condition in which an erection is initially obtained, but quickly lost after insertion into the vagina.

Stress incontinence: Characterized by a small loss of urine following some sudden strain on the body such as coughing or laughing.

Support group: Voluntary group of individuals who meet periodically to exchange information and to provide mutual comfort in connection with some medical problem. Various prostate cancer and impotence support groups exist for men and their families.

Suprapubic prostatectomy: Prostatectomy in which a surgical incision is made through the abdomen at a point above where the penis enters the body, bypassing the bladder as the cut is extended to the prostate.

T

Testicles: Two glands located inside the scrotum that produce sperm and sex hormones, including testosterone. While the plural is "testes," "testicles" is used in this book according to common current usage.

Testosterone: Principal male sex hormone produced largely in the testicles and in lesser quantities in the adrenal gland. Testosterone stimulates male sexual characteristics as well as the growth of benign and malignant prostatic tissue.

Three-piece inflatable penile implant: Most complex and generally most effective penile prosthesis consisting of cylindrical elements implanted inside the penis, a pump and valve mechanism implanted inside the scrotum, and a reservoir for hydraulic fluid implanted in the lower abdomen.

Transrectal ultrasound of the prostate (TRUS): Test procedure using ultrasound to observe and diagnose prostate enlargement. *See* "Ultrasound."

Transurethral hyperthermia (TH): New treatment for benign prostate enlargement; heat generated by a microwave transmitter alleviates urinary obstruction.

Transurethral incision of the prostate (TUIP): New treatment for benign prostate enlargement; a series of small cuts is made inside the urethra to alleviate urinary obstruction.

Transurethral resection of the prostate (TURP): Form of prostatectomy used with benign prostate enlargement; excess prostate tissue interfering with proper urination is removed with a device known as a resectoscope inserted through the penis.

Transurethral ultrasound-guided laser prostatectomy (TULIP): New prostatectomy technique used with benign prostate enlargement; a laser beam guided by an ultrasound image removes excess prostate tissue that interferes with normal urination.

Trichomonas vaginalis: Microorganism that causes vaginal infections in women and can spread in men to the urethra and prostate. Also, trick.

Tuberculosis: Serious and once-common infectious disease now making a comeback as a consequence of the AIDS epidemic. Tuberculosis can cause a form of prostatitis.

Tumor: Body mass caused by abnormal cell growth. Tumors can be benign or malignant.

U

Ultrasound: High-frequency sound waves used for medical diagnosis and treatment. In an ultrasound scan (or sonogram), sound waves reflected by internal organs produce computer-enhanced images. Ultrasound is also used to treat prostate enlargement. *See* "transurethral ultrasound."

Ureter: Tube that carries urine produced in each kidney to the bladder.

Urethra: Tube starting at the base of the bladder and passing through the penis that carries urine and semen outside the body.

Urgency (or urge) incontinence: Characterized by sudden contraction of the bladder, a condition commonly caused by infection or neurological disease.

Urinalysis: Series of tests performed on a patient's urine sample; important in diagnosing prostatitis, urinary infections, bladder and kidney cancer, diabetes, and other conditions.

Urinary retention: Critical medical emergency associated with benign prostate enlargement; quantities of urine back up into the bladder causing damage to the bladder and kidneys. Sometimes fatal if not treated immediately.

Urologist: Physician specializing in urological disorders. Although urologists treat both men and women, they are sometimes referred to as the "male doctor," owing to their important role in treating the unique physical problems of men.

Urology: Branch of medicine dealing with disorders of the urinary system in men and women and disorders of the genital (sex) organs in men.

V

Vaginal yeast infection: Vaginal infection in women caused by microscopic yeast organisms. Yeast infections can be sexually transmitted and can cause a form of prostatitis.

Vas deferens: Two ducts that transport semen from each of the testicles. The vas deferens join into a single duct near the prostate and urethra, which then connects to the ejaculatory duct.

Vasectomy: Surgical procedure in which the two vas deferens of a male are severed and tied off to achieve voluntary sterility. A vasectomy does not make a man impotent.

Vegan: Strict vegetarian who will not eat meat or any other animal product, including milk, cheese, and eggs. A vegan may develop a zinc deficiency, important to a healthy prostate.

Virus: Group of microorganisms smaller than bacteria that cannot be seen with a conventional microscope. Viruses are large protein molecules that can multiply only by attacking living cells.

Vitamin: Complex organic chemical compound found in most natural food products essential in the diet of humans and other animals. Vitamins A, C, and E appear most relevant to the healthy prostate.

Voiding studies: Group of studies used to diagnose and evaluate benign prostate enlargement, involving observation and measurement of a patient's urinary flow and related characteristics.

W

White cells: Cells found in the bloodstream that protect the body from disease by attacking bacteria or by producing antibodies. Pus, a yellowish material, is formed when white cells attack bacteria and is an indication of prostatitis and other infections.

X

X rays: Subatomic high energy particles of short wave length that can penetrate body tissues. X rays produce photographic images for diagnostic purposes. In radiation therapy, they destroy cancerous growth.

Z

Zinc: Metallic mineral essential in the diets of all animals, including humans. Normally, the prostate contains a high concentration of zinc, so there is good evidence that zinc is important to prostate health.

Prostate Medications

The following medications are mentioned elsewhere in this book. Each entry in-cludes manufacturers' proprietary brand names, generic equivalents or the generic names of active ingredients, information on the most serious or relevant side ef-fects, and important precautions and other comments. Drugs readily available as generics are indicated.

Brand Name	Generic Name or Generic Ingredients	Side Effects/ Comments

Prostatitis, Prostatosis, and Prostatodynia

Advil	Ibuprofen, pseudoephedrine	Anti-inflammatory. May cause nervous-ness, dizziness, and insomnia. Do not take if aspirin sensitive. Use with caution in patients with BPH. Available in other brand names or generically.
Ambihar	Niridazole	Antischistosomiasis drug. May cause headaches, dizziness, nervousness, and gastrointestinal problems.
Amcil	Ampicillin	Antibiotic for prostatitis. May cause gastrointestinal problems and

Brand Name	Generic Name or Generic Ingredients	Side Effects/ Comments
		allergic reactions. Available in other brand names and generically.
Amoxil	Amoxicillin	Antibiotic for gonorrheal prostatitis. May cause gastrointestinal problems and allergic reactions. Should not be used by patients with history of allergic reactions to any form of penicillin. Available in other brand names and generically.
Ansaid	Fluorbiprofen	Anti-inflammatory. May cause gastro-intestinal or nervous system problems. Use with caution in patients with kidney or liver disorders.
Bactrim	Trimethoprim, sulfamethoxazole	Antibacterial. May cause allergic reactions, gastrointestinal problems, blood disorders, headaches, and depression. A sulfa drug that should be used with caution in patients with impaired kidney or liver function, asthma, or who take anticoagulants such as Coumarin (warfarin).
Bicillin	Procaine penicillin	Antibiotic for gonorrheal prostatitis. May cause allergic reactions. Should not be used by patients with history of sensitivity to any type of penicillin. Available in other brand names.
Cipro	Ciprofloxacin	Fluoroquinolone drug for treating bacterial prostatitis.

Brand Name	Generic Name or Generic Ingredients	Side Effects/ Comments
Flagyl	Metronidazole	For trichomonas infections. May cause convulsions, numbness in extremities, and nausea. Use with caution in patients with liver disorders or who take anticoagulants. *Absolutely no alcohol use while taking drug.*
Floxin	Ofloxacin	Experimental fluoroquinolone drug for treating bacterial prostatitis.
INH Tablets	Isoniazid	Antituberculosis drug (taken in combination with other drugs). May cause numbness in extremities or liver problems.
Myambutol	Ethambutol	Antituberculosis drug (taken in combination with other drugs). May cause problems with vision. Patients using drug should be monitored frequently for eye disorders.
Noroxin	Norfloxacin	Fluoroquinolone drug for treating bacterial prostatitis.
Nizoral	Ketonazole	Antifungal drug for yeast infections of the prostate. May cause nausea and vomiting.
Nystatin	Nystatin	Antifungal drug for yeast infections of the prostate. May cause gastrointestinal problems.
PAS	Aminosalicylic acid	Antituberculosis drug (taken in

Brand Name	Generic Name or Generic Ingredients	Side Effects/ Comments
		combination with other drugs). May cause gastrointestinal problems. Should not be taken by patients with stomach ulcers or who are aspirin sensitive.
Septra	Trimethoprim, sulfamethoxazole	Antibacterial. May cause allergic reactions, gastrointestinal problems, blood disorders, headaches, and depression. A sulfa drug to be used with caution in patients with impaired kidney or liver function, asthma, or who take anticoagulants such as Coumarin (warfarin).
	Streptomycin	Antituberculosis drug (taken in combination with other drugs). Extended use may cause deafness or hearing problems.
Terramycin	Tetracycline	Antibiotic for treating chlamydia infections of the prostate. May cause gastrointestinal problems, skin rashes, and allergic reactions. Available in other brand names or generically.
Thiomicid	Thiacetazone	Antituberculosis drug (taken in combination with other drugs). May cause skin rashes, vomiting, dizziness, or loss of appetite.
Vibramycin	Doxycycline	Antibiotic for treating chlamydia infections of the prostate. May cause skin rashes, gastrointestinal problems, and

Brand Name	Generic Name or Generic Ingredients	Side Effects/ Comments
		allergic reactions. Available under other brand names.

Benign Prostatic Hyperplasia (BPH)

Brand Name	Generic Name or Generic Ingredients	Side Effects/ Comments
Cardura	Doxazosin mesylate	Relaxes a type of muscle in the prostate, to improve urine flow. Should improve flow within one to two weeks. Also used to treat high blood pressure. Side effects include dizziness, fatigue, and edema.
Dibenzyline	Phenoxybenzamine	Experimental drug for BPH with alpha adrenergic-blocking properties.
Estrace	Estradiol (Estrogen)	Female hormone for blocking testosterone. May cause loss of libido and breast enlargement. Available in other brand names.
Eulexin	Flutamine	Antiandrogen drug for controlling output of testosterone by the adrenal gland. May cause hot flashes, loss of libido, impotence, and gastrointestinal problems.
Hytrin	Terazosin	Drug for treating high blood pressure with alpha adrenergic-blocking properties. Under investigation for treatment of benign prostate enlargement. May cause dizziness, headaches, tiredness, nasal congestion, and abnormally low blood pressure.

Brand Name	Generic Name or Generic Ingredients	Side Effects/ Comments
Minipress	Prazosin	Drug for treating high blood pressure with alpha adrenergic-blocking properties. Under investigation for treatment of benign prostate enlargement. May cause dizziness, headaches, tiredness, and sudden loss of consciousness.
Proscar	Finasteride	Testosterone-controlling drug approved in 1992 for general use in treating BPH. Reversible impotence is a side effect in a small percentage of users. Possible danger to male fetuses in women made pregnant by men taking drug.

Prostate Cancer

Casodex	Bicalutamide	An antiandrogen drug blocking production of testosterone in adrenal gland. Side effects can include hot flashes, pain, diarrhea, and constipation.
CPA	Cyproterone	A progestin (not FDA approved).
Cytadren	Aminoglutithamide	Antiandrogen drug for blocking output of testosterone by adrenal gland. Taken in combination with hydrocortisone. May cause nausea, drowsiness, and skin rash. For use in a hospital setting.
Estrace	Estriadiol (Estrogen)	Female hormone to block testosterone. May cause loss of libido and breast enlargement. Available in other brand names.

Brand Name	Generic Name or Generic Ingredients	Side Effects/ Comments
Eulexin	Flutamide	Antiandrogen drug for blocking output of testosterone by adrenal gland. May cause hot flashes, loss of libido, impotence, and gastrointestinal problems.
Lupron	Leuprolide acetate	Testosterone-blocking drug used in luteinizing hormone-releasing hormone therapy (LHRH). May cause hot flashes, edema, general pain, gastrointestinal problems, and tiredness.
Megase	Megastrol (MGA)	A progestin or steroidal antiandrogen. Blocks the effects of androgens. No heart complications, but effective for a limited time.
Zoladex	Goserelin acetate	Antiandrogen drug blocking action of adrenal glands. May cause hot flashes and sexual dysfunction. Use with caution in patients with urinary obstructions and spinal cord compression.

Impotence

Caverject	Prostaglandin E_1	Penile injection of drug may result in adequate erection. For use only under urologist's supervision. Improper use may cause priapism or penile scarring.
Cerebid	Papaverine	Penile injection of drug may result in adequate erection. For use only under urologist's supervision. Improper use may cause priapism or penile scarring. Available under other brand names.

Brand Name	Generic Name or Generic Ingredients	Side Effects/ Comments
Regitine	Phentolamine	Penile injection of drug may result in adequate erection. For use only under urologist's supervision. Improper use may cause priapism or penile scarring.
Desyrel	Trazadone	Oral drug for treating impotence by improving function of the smooth muscles of the penis. Used in higher dosages as an antidepressant. Impotence patients should never take more than the prescribed dosage.
Viagra	Sildenafil	Oral drug for treating erectile dysfunction by increasing blood flow and erectile stimulation. May cause headaches, indigestion, and color/brightness visionary disturbances. Should not be taken by patients with severe kidney or liver failure, rare disease retinitis pigmentosa of the eye, or using nitroglycerin or nitrates.
Yocon	Yohimbine	Drug with apparent aphrodisiac properties. May cause elevated blood pressure, rapid heart rate, irritability, tremor, dizziness, headache, and nausea. Available in other brand names.

Where to Get Prostate Information and Support

A growing number of organizations provide information and support to men with prostate problems and to their family members. Here is a list of known sources of help and assistance:

General Information on Prostate Problems

American Foundation for Urologic Disease, Inc.

The American Foundation for Urologic Disease, Inc., Baltimore, Maryland, is a non-profit group organized to educate the general public on urological problems and to encourage research in the field. Although the foundation emphasizes prostate cancer, information is also available on benign prostate enlargement, prostate infections, and other problems. The Foundation engages in a number of educational, lobbying, and support activities. It publishes the magazine *Family Urology*.

For information, write or call:

> American Foundation for Urologic Disease
> 300 West Pratt Street
> Suite 401
> Baltimore, MD 21201
> 1-800-242-2383

American Urological Association

The American Urological Association, Baltimore, Maryland, founded 1902, is the principal professional society representing over 6,000 physicians who specialize in urologic disorders. The association publishes the authoritative *Journal of Urology,* holds scientific conferences, and supports the activities of eight regional sections representing members throughout the United States, Canada, Mexico, Central America, the Pacific, and the Caribbean. For information, call or write:

> American Urological Association
> 1120 North Charles Street
> Baltimore, MD 21201
> (410) 727-1100
> www.auanet.org

National Kidney and Urologic Diseases Information Clearinghouse

This division of the National Institutes of Health is a source of scientific research and general information about medical treatments for prostatitis and BPH, but not prostate cancer.

> National Kidney and Urologic Diseases Clearinghouse
> Box NKUDIC
> 3 Information Way
> Betheseda, MD 20892-3580
> (301) 654-4415; (301) 468-6345
> www.niddk.nih.gov

Prostate Cancer Education Council

> Prostate Cancer Education Council
> 1180 Avenue of the Americas
> New York, NY 10036
> (212) 221-3300
> http://www.cancercare.org

Prostatitis

The Prostatitis Foundation

The Prostatitis Foundation distributes educational literature, maintains a volunteer telephone support bank, and advocates for research on this common male disease.

> The Prostatitis Foundation
> Information Distribution Center
> Parkway Business Center
> 2029 Ireland Grove Road
> Bloomington, IL 61704

World Wide Web addresses:

> http://www.prostate.org
> http://www.fullfeed.com/prosfnd/

Benign Prostate Hyperplasia (BPH)

American Medical Systems

American Medical Systems, a leading manufacturer of medical devices, including balloon dilatation equipment, penile implants, and artificial sphincters, provides free information to the public on BPH. For information, write or call:

> Information Center
> American Medical Systems
> 11001 Bren Road East
> Minnetonka, Minnesota 55343
> 1-800-543-9632

Merck & Co.

The major pharmaceutical manufacturer Merck & Co. offers free information to customers and health care professionals. For information on the BPH drug Proscar, or any other Merck product, write or call:

> Merck & Co., Inc.
> West Point, PA 19486
> 1-800-672-6372
> www.merck.com

Prostate Cancer

American Cancer Society

The American Cancer Society, Atlanta, Georgia, founded 1913, provides information and a wide variety of other useful assistance including, in some instances, financial aid for prostate and other cancers. The Society operates through 58 regional and 3,000 local groups.

For information, write or call:

> American Cancer Society
> 1599 Clifton Road
> Atlanta, GA 30329
> 1-800-ACS-2345
> www. cancer. org

National Cancer Institute
Office of Cancer Communications
Building 31, Room 10A24
Bethesda, MD 20892

The Prostate Health Council
c/o American Foundation for Urologic Disease, Inc.
300 West Pratt Street, Suite 401
Baltimore, MD 21201
1-800-242-2383

The Geddings Osbon Foundation
P.O. Box 1593
Augusta, GA 30903
1-800-433-9017

American Prostate Society
(410) 859-3735
http://www.ameripros.org

Cap Cure (Association for the Cure of Cancer of the Prostate)
1-800-757-CURE
http://www.capcure.org

The Mathews Foundation For Prostate Cancer Research
1-800-234-6284
http://www.mathews.org

National Institutes of Health

The National Institutes of Health (NIH), Bethesda, Maryland, a unit of the U.S. government, operates a free service providing cancer information. Persons calling an 800 number are automatically put in contact with the nearest regional Cancer Information Service. Information available on prostate cancer includes booklets and a computer printout of the status of the latest clinical trials of drugs and other cancer treatments being conducted under the auspices of the National Cancer Institute. Individuals with a prostate cancer problem are encouraged to mention this clinical trial data to their physicians.

For information, call: 1-800-4-CANCER
rex.nci.nih.gov

Patient Advocates for Advanced Cancer Treatments (PAACT)

PAACT is a nonprofit membership organization, incorporated in 1987, which lends support and provides information on advanced prostate cancer treatments. Members receive a monthly newsletter, the *Prostate Cancer Report*, and access to a computerized telephone service that offers dialogs on prostate cancer. PAACT's advocacy role has included aggressive efforts to improve and accelerate approval procedures for new drugs by the U.S. Food and Drug Administration.

For information, write or call:

PAACT, Inc.
P. O. Box 141695
Grand Rapids, MI 49514-1695
(616) 453-1477
www.osz.com/paact

Prostate Cancer Support Network

The Prostate Cancer Support Network, a division of the American Foundation for Urologic Disease, will assist in setting up local US-Too and other prostate cancer support groups with educational materials and other types of assistance.

Prostate Cancer Education Council
230 Park Avenue South
New York, NY 10003

Prostate Cancer Support Network
300 W. Pratt Street, Suite 401
Baltimore, MD 21201
1-800-828-7866

National Hospice Organization

The National Hospice Organization can help locate a hospice within a local area.

National Hospice Organization
1901 North Moore Street, Suite 901
Arlington, VA 22209
1-800-658-8898
www.nho.org

Theragenics Corporation

Therogenics Corporation, Norcross, Georgia, is a major manufacturer of radioactive pellets or "seeds" used in interstitial radiation therapy treatment of prostate cancer. The company provides an information service regarding radiation therapy and Therogenics's products.

For information, write or call:

Therogenics Corporation
5325 Oak Brook Parkway
Norcross, GA 30093
1-800-458-4372 or (770) 381-8338
www.therogenics.com

US-TOO, INTERNATIONAL

US-TOO INTERNATIONAL is a network of support groups for men who have had prostate cancer and their families. There are more than four hundred US-TOO chapters in all fifty states, and several active chapters in Canada, Australia, Turkey, Germany, and England. US-TOO publishes the US-TOO Prostate Cancer Communicator, a quarterly newsletter and provides information on prostate cancer treatments. To receive information, including the location of the nearest US-TOO chapter and its coordinator, write or call:

US-TOO, INTERNATIONAL
930 North York Road, Suite 50
Hinsdale, IL 60521-2993
1-800-808-7866
www.ustoo.com

Impotence

Men with impotence problems resulting from prostate surgery or any other cause, and their partners, may obtain information and support by contacting the Impotence Institute of America, Washington, D.C., the nearest local chapter of Impotence Anonymous, or the American Medical Systems Information Center, Minneapolis, Minnesota.

Impotence Institute of America/Impotence Anonymous

The Impotence Institute of America, Inc., founded 1983, is a national nonprofit organization representing the interests of men with impotence problems, physicians with a special interest in the impotence field, and private companies manufacturing products for treating impotence. The Institute supports its affiliated self-help support group, Impotence Anonymous. About seventy-five chapters are located in most major metropolitan centers.

Individuals needing assistance may obtain free publications, referrals to appropriate physicians in their areas, and the location of the nearest chapter of Impotence Anonymous by writing or telephoning:

> Impotence Institute of America, Inc.
> P.O. Box 410
> Bowie, MD 20718-0410
> 1-800-669-1603 or (301) 262-2400
>
> Impotence World Association
> 1-800-669-1603

You may also obtain information and assistance by contacting the nearest Impotence Institute of America regional medical advisers, listed below:

Arkansas

Steven K. Wilson, M.D.
2015 Chestnut
Van Buren, AR 72956
(501) 474-1225

Arizona – New Mexico

Michael A. Chasin, M.D.
Consultants in Urology, Ltd.
1500 South Dobson Road, Suite 315
Mesa, AZ 85202
(602) 834-0269

Northern California

Robert S. Safran, M.D.
444 34th Street
Oakland, CA 94609
(510) 420-8114

Southern California – Southern Nevada

Stephen M. Auerbach, M.D.
400 Newport Center Drive, Suite 50
Newport Beach, CA 92662
(714) 644-7200

Florida

Richard L. Fein, M.D.
Fein & Winton Associates
12900 NE 17th Avenue, Suite 301
North Miami, FL 33181
(305) 891-5060

Georgia – Alabama

Steven Morganstern, M.D.
Morganstern Urology Clinic
3280 Howell Mill Road, Suite 125-West
Atlanta, GA 30327
(404) 352-8220
1-800-652-5644

Illinois – Indiana

Terry Mason, M.D.
Attention: Tom Bleser
8541 South State, Suite 9
Chicago, IL 60619
(312) 846-7000

Maryland – Delaware

Myron I. Murdock, M.D.
7500 Hanover Parkway, Suite 206
Greenbelt, MD 20770
(301) 441-8900

North Dakota – South Dakota – Montana – Wyoming – Idaho

Manuel Neto, M.D.
P.O. Box 40
1500 24th Avenue, SW
Minot, ND 58702
(701) 852-6386

New Jersey

Matis A. Fermaglich, M.D.
865 Teaneck Road
Teaneck, NJ 07666-4513
(201) 837-0606

New York – Connecticut

E. Douglas Whitehead, M.D.
785 Park Avenue
New York, NY 10021
(212) 879-3131

Oklahoma – Kansas

James R. Leach, M.D.
1725 East 19th Street, Suite 801
Tulsa, OK 74104
(918) 749-8765

Pennsylvania

Alan N. Fleischer, M.D.
Urology Associates
200 North 13th Street, Suite 201
Reading, PA 19604
(215) 372-2351

Texas

David F. Mobley, M.D.
920 Frostwood, Suite 610
Houston, TX 77024
(713) 932-1819

Virginia – Washington, D.C.

David Schwartz, M.D.
5252 Dawes Avenue
Alexandria, VA 22311
(703) 998-7333

Information Center, American Medical Systems

American Medical Systems, a leading manufacturer of medical devices, including equipment for balloon dilatation, penile implants, and artificial sphincters, offers free information to the general public in connection with impotence and incontinence. See reference in BPH section above.

Information Center
American Medical Systems
Minneapolis, MN 55440
1-800-543-9632

Impotence and Incontinence — Sexual Problems

American Association of Sex Educators,
Counselors and Therapists
435 North Michigan Avenue
Suite 1717
Chicago, IL 60611
(312) 644-0828

Impotence Information Center

This informational clearinghouse is sponsored by American Medical Systems. It produces the publication, *Impotence Help in the USA*, available upon request, and will furnish a custom list of urologists who specialize in treating impotence in a patient's local area.

Impotence Information Center
American Medical Systems
11001 Bren Road East
Minnetonka, Minnesota 55343
1-800-543-9632

Impotence Institute of America
P.O. Box 410
Bowie, Maryland 20718-0410
1-800-669-1603

Incontinence

Individuals with incontinence problems resulting from prostate surgery or some other cause can obtain assistance by contacting Help for Incontinent People, Union, South Carolina, or an information service provided by a major manufacturer of incontinence products. You also should check the health and fitness section of your newspaper to see if any local hospital or medical group is providing information and assistence.

Help for Incontinent People

Help for Incontinent People (HIP), founded 1982, is a nonprofit organization providing information and services throughout North America to both men and women with incontinence problems. Interested individuals may join HIP for an annual membership fee of $15. The annual fee includes four issues of the newsletter, *The HIP Report*; a personal response service for individuals with specific questions on incontinence problems; and the *Resource Guide to Continence Products and Services*. Other services include the Continence Reference Service, which provides names of health professionals specializing in incontinence in your state, informational pamphlets, and audio/visual programs which are available for a modest charge.

For further information write or phone:

> Help for Incontinent People (HIP)
> P.O. Box 8310
> Spartanburg, SC 29305
> 1-800-BLADDER
> www.nafc.org
>
> Home Delivery Incontinence
> 1-800-538-1036
> http://www.hdisnet.com

Information Center, American Medical Systems

American Medical Systems, a leading manufacturer of medical devices, including equipment for balloon dilatation, penile implants, and artificial urinary sphincters offers a free information service. See reference in BHP section above.

Kimberly-Clark Corporation

Kimberly-Clark Corporation is a leading manufacturer of adult incontinence care products. You are probably aware of the company's television commercials for its Depend absorbent products line featuring the actress, June Allyson. As a free service, the company provides information and responds to specific questions on incontinence in general as well as on its incontinence products. For information write or call:

> Kimberly-Clark Home Health Care
> P. O. Box 2020
> Neenah, WI 54957-2020
> Telephone (weekdays between 9 AM and 3 PM CST)
> In Wisconsin: 1-800-242-6463
> Outside Wisconsin: 1-800-558-6423
> www.depend.com

Procter & Gamble

The Procter & Gamble Co., Cincinnati, Ohio, a well-known consumer products manufacturer, provides information and free samples of the company's adult incontinence products, which are sold under the name Attend. Write or call:

> The Procter & Gamble Co.
> Procter & Gamble Plaza
> Cincinnati, OH 45202
> (General information): 1-800-432-4000
> (Product sample): 1-800-4-ATTEND
> www.pg.com

The Simon Foundation

The Simon Foundation, Wilmette, Illinois, an organization with over 80,000 members, conducts research and provides educational services on incontinence. For information, write or call:

> The Simon Foundation
> Box 815
> Wilmette, IL 60091
> 1-800-23-SIMON

Other Prostate Resources

Many local hospitals and medical groups offer informational seminars, sponsor support groups, or provide other forms of assistance in connection with prostate problems. Check the health section of your local newspaper, especially on weekends, for announcements and articles on these activities.

Patients often express an interest in participating in clinical trials of new prostate drugs. If your physician does not have information on drug trials, try calling the help line numbers of Merck & Co. and the National Institutes of Health (listed previously) or contact the department of urology at your nearest medical school. You should be aware that in clinical trials some patients do receive placebos, not the new drug being tested.

On-Line Information

More and more, on-line discussion newsgroups are sources for useful information. Apply the same standards in assessing information you receive from electronic sources that you would apply anyplace else, such as in reading a book or watching a news broadcast. A few electronic resources are listed below:

Internet Newsgroups:

> sci.med.prostate.bph
> sci.med.prostate.cancer
> sci.med.prostate.prostatitis
> sci.med.diseases.cancer
> sci.med.nutrition
> sci.med.prostate.cancer
> alt.support
> alt.support.cancer
> alt.support.prostate.cancer

alt.support.depression
alt.health.policy.drug-approval
alt.med.immunology
misc.health.alternative

World Wide Web Pages:

http://www.prostate.org
http://www.parsec.it/summit/pO.htm
http://www.vix.com/pub/men/health/articles/prostatitis.html
http://rattler.cameron.edu/prostate/html
http://www.secapl.com/prostate/top/html
http://www.cancer.med.umich.edu/prostcan.html
http://cancer.med.upenn.edu/
www.mediXperts.com

Note: if you have trouble with any of the above, an e-mail address where you can get more information is:

prostate-request@sjuvm.stjohns.edu

Indexes:

CanSearch: Online Guide to Cancer Resources
http://www.cansearch.org/canserch/canserch.htm

Links to Cancer Institutes and Research Centers
http://seidata.com/~marriage/rcancer.html

Medicine OnLine
http://www.meds.com/

Quick Information About Cancer for Patients and Their Families
http://asa.ugl.lib.umich.edu/chdocs/cancer/CANCERGUIDE.HTML

Government Servers:

National Cancer Institute/CancerNet
http://www.nci.nih.gov/

National Institutes of Health WWW Server
http://www.nih.gov/

National Library of Medicine
http://www.nlm.nih.gov/

Alternative Medicine Home Page
http://www.pitt.edu/~cbw/altm.html

CancerGuide
http://cancerguide.org/

Cancer News on the Net
http://www.cancernews.com

CenterWatch: Clinical Trials Listing Service
http://www.centerwatch.com/

HealthGate
http://www.healthgate.com

International Cancer Alliance
http://www2.ari.net/icare/

Prostate Cancer InfoLink
http://www.comed.com/prostate/

Grateful Med
http://igm.nlm.nih.gov

PubMed
http://www.ncbi.nlm.nih.gov/pubmed/

National Library of Medicine
http://www.nlm.nih.gov/

The Combined Health Information Database
http://chid.nih.gov

Web Sites/Clinics and Research Centers

Albert Einstein Cancer Center
http://www.ca.aecom.yu.edu/

Cedars-Sinai Comprehensive Cancer Center
http://csccc.com/

City of Hope National Cancer Center
http://www.cityofhope.org/

Frederick Cancer Research and Development Center
http://www.ncifcrf.gov/

Fox Chase Cancer Center
http://www.fccc.edu/

H. Lee Moffitt Cancer Center
http://daisy.moffitt.usf.edu

M.D. Anderson Cancer Center/University of Texas
http://utmdacc.uth.tmc.edu/

Memorial Sloan-Kettering Cancer Center
http://www.mskcc.org

The Cancer Institute of New Jersey
http://www-cinj.umdnj.edu/

University of California San Francisco Cancer Center
http://cc.ucsf.edu/

University of Michigan Comprehensive Cancer Center
http://www.cancer.med.umich.edu/

Cancer-Related Web Sites in Spanish

New York Online Access to Health
http://www.noah.cuny.edu/

The March: Unamonos Para Derrotar Al Cancer (National Coalition
For Cancer Survivorship)
http://www.themarch.org/

The Mautner Project for Lesbians With Cancer
http://www.sirius.com/~edisol/mautner/spanish.html

Public, University, and Medical Libraries

In addition to public libraries, university, hospital, or medical school libraries can sometimes be used to find books or articles about cancer. However, not all hospital and medical school libraries are open to the public, so it is advisable to call and ask about their policy and to find out whether they have copies of the journals or books you might want.

The National Library of Medicine
8600 Rockville Pike
Bethesda, MD 20894
1-888-346-3656 or (301) 594-5983

Diagnosing BPH

Is It Possible That You Have BPH?

Write down the answers to the following seven questions. Give yourself a score of 0 for never, 1 for less than 20 percent of the time, 2 for less than 50 percent of the time, 3 for about 50 percent of the time, 4 for more than 50 percent of the time, and 5 for almost all the time. Add the appropriate number of times for Question 7 to the total of the first six questions to calculate your score.

1. Over the past month, how often have you had a sensation of not emptying your bladder completely after you finished urinating?
2. Over the past month, how often have you had to urinate less than two hours after you finished urinating?
3. Over the past month, how often have you found that you stopped and started again several times when you urinated?
4. Over the past month, how often have you found it difficult to postpone urination?
5. Over the past month, how often have you had a weak urinary stream?
6. Over the past month, how often have you had to push or strain to begin urination?
7. Over the past month, how many times did you most typically get up to urinate from the time you went to bed at night until the time you got up in the morning?

Scores ranging from 0–7 are considered mild, from 8–19 moderate, from 20–35 severe. The American Urological Association notes that the higher the score, the more likely you will need treatment for BPH.

SOURCE: THE AMERICAN UROLOGICAL ASSOCIATION

General Questions to Ask Your Doctor

These are questions suggested by the American Cancer Society.

Diagnosis

1. Has my cancer spread (metasized) to other parts of my body?
2. What stage is my cancer?
3. Can you tell if this is a fast-growing type of prostate cancer, or a slow-growing type? (What is the Gleason score and ploidy type?)

Tests

1. What tests will I have done?
2. When should I expect the results from these tests?
3. What will these tests tell me about my cancer?
4. How long after I have these tests will I know the results?
5. Who will call me with the results of these tests? Or, should I call to obtain the results?
6. If I need to get copies of my records, scans, or X rays, who should I contact?

Physician

1. Did you consult with anyone before determining the diagnosis?
2. What will their role be in my treatment?
3. How many physicians will be involved in my care? Who are they? What are their roles?

4. Who will be the physician in charge of coordinating all the rest of my physicians?
5. What other health care professionals can I expect to be involved in my care?
6. Do you recommend surgery? If so, what are my options involving surgery?
7. Is nerve-sparing surgery possible in my case?
8. What percentage (approximately) of the nerve-conserving surgeries you have done have been successful?
9. Would you give me the telephone number of two other patients?

Treatment

1. What is the standard treatment for my type of prostate cancer?
2. What is the prognosis for my type of prostate cancer with standard treatment?
3. Are there any other treatments that might be appropriate for my type of prostate cancer?
4. What treatment do you recommend? Based on what?
5. What are the risks or benefits of the treatment you are recommending?
6. Am I a good candidate for a radiation seed implant where the seeds are left in?
7. Am I a good candidate for a radiation seed implant where the seeds are inserted and removed?
8. Who would you recommend I talk to about the different treatments?
9. What doctors do you know who are experts at the seed implant radiation techniques?
10. What percentage of patients usually respond to this treatment?
11. How long does each treatment last?
12. How long will the entire course of therapy last?
13. How often will I be treated?
14. What type of results should I expect to see with the treatment?
15. Will there be tests during my treatment to determine if it is working?
16. Where will I receive my treatment?
17. How will I receive my treatment? Is it a pill? an injection?
18. What will it feel like to get treated?
19. Can someone accompany me to my treatment?

20. Can I drive to and from my appointments?
21. Can I stay alone after my treatments, or do I need to have someone stay with me?
22. Will I have to be in the hospital to get my treatments?
23. Who will administer my treatments?
24. How often, during treatment, will I see a physician? the nurse?

Clinical Trials

1. Are there any clinical trials or research being done on my type of prostate cancer?
2. Are you involved in clinical trials?
3. Would I be a candidate for clinical research if it is a treatment option for me?
4. Where can I find out more about research on prostate cancer?
5. Is there anyone else in the area that is involved in research that I might contact to discuss my prostate cancer?
6. What will happen if I decide not to be treated?
7. How quickly must I decide about my treatment?

Economics

1. How do I find out what portion of the treatment my insurance company will cover?
2. Is there someone in your office (or facility) who assists patients with questions about insurance? Who would that be?
3. If my insurance does not pay for a particular treatment or medication that might be beneficial to me, will you choose an alternate treatment? What if it is less effective?
4. Do you have access to pharmaceutical patient assistance programs I could access if I cannot afford a particular medication or my insurance will not pay for a particular medication?
5. Who can I talk to about getting treatment if I do not have insurance?

Support

1. Do you provide any literature that suggests ways to tell my family of my illness?

2. Are you willing to speak with my wife (or other family members) about my prostate cancer and my treatment?
3. Are there support groups for prostate cancer?
4. For my family and friends?
5. Is there a social worker here I could talk to?
6. How do I access a dietitian if I have nutritional concerns or difficulties?
7. Do I need to be on a special diet?
8. If I can have sex after my treatment, will my partner be at risk in any way?
9. What type of precautions do I need to take?
10. Who do I call if I have any emergency medical situation during my treatment, or shortly afterward?
11. What are the telephone numbers I should have in order to reach you? the nurse? the hospital?

Side Effects

What are the side effects of this treatment?

— Nausea
— Vomiting
— Hair loss
— Low blood cell counts (anemia: low red-blood-cell count, neutropenia: low count of one type of white-blood cell, low platelets, etc.)
— Diarrhea/constipation
— Skin changes
— Incontinence
— Impotence
— Pain
— Sores along the digestive tract
— Taste changes
— Neuropathy (damage to nerves)
— Slow heart beat
— Irregular heart beat
— Fatigue

1. When might these side effects occur?
2. Could these side effects be life-threatening?

3. How long will the side effects last?
4. What can/will be done to prevent these side effects or reduce their possibility?
5. When might these side effects occur?
6. Could these side effects be life-threatening?
7. How long will the side effects last?

Supportive Therapies

1. What treatments are available to manage these side effects?
2. Are these support therapies available and appropriate for me?
3. What should I do if I have side effects?
4. Who do I call if I have severe side effects?
5. Will a reduction or delay reduce my chances of being cured?
6. Are there any medications I should not take while I'm going through treatment?
7. Are there any activities I should or should not do following treatment?
8. How soon after treatment can I go back to work?

Index